Juice Cleanse Recipes

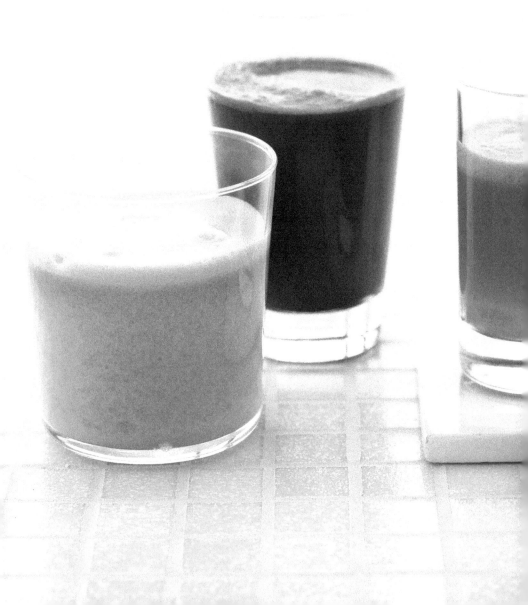

Juice Cleanse Recipes

JUICING DETOX PLANS TO
REVITALIZE HEALTH AND ENERGY

MENDOCINO
PRESS

Contents

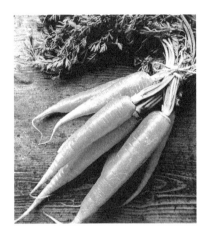

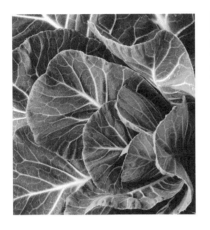

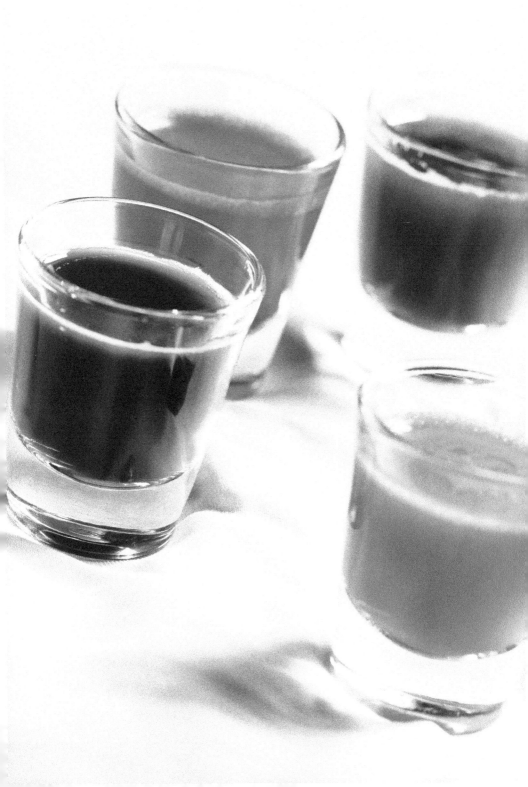

Introduction

Ask the average person about his or her number one health goal and the answer is almost always weight loss. It seems most people have a constant desire to lose five, ten, or even twenty (or more) pounds. They try every type of diet plan to reach this goal, too: low-carb, gluten-free, Paleo—you name it.

But the best approach to obtaining and maintaining your ideal weight may require only a drinking glass. Fruit and vegetable juices can offer almost everything you need to change your eating habits, clear your body of built-up toxins, and rejuvenate your natural detox system so you may finally begin to burn fat, lose weight, and, most important, keep weight off.

Fruits and vegetables contain all the essential vitamins, minerals, enzymes, and nutrients you need to lose weight. The problem is that most Americans do not consume nearly enough. Instead, the standard American diet consists of high-fat and high-calorie meals and processed food that not only contribute to weight gain but also prevent people from ever losing excess weight.

A short-term juice cleanse, however, is the ideal method for getting more fruits and vegetables into your daily diet. It also helps you break the cycle of poor eating habits and introduce new, healthier ones. And juices are so easy to make—all you need is a juicer. With so many flavors, you can create an almost endless variety of beverages that are healthful and free of any commercial processing.

This book provides a real diet plan. It shows how juicing can play a specific role in your health and well-being, with a detailed explanation of how a juice cleanse works and what it's designed to accomplish. This book also explains how fruits and vegetables can help with weight loss, which ones are ideal for juicing, and more specifically, how a structured juice cleanse lasting one, three, five, or seven days may change your eating habits and help you achieve lasting weight loss.

You'll also learn how to properly prepare for a cleanse, and you'll be provided with tips to help you succeed during the cleansing process and after. With 125 exciting and flavorful juice recipes, you can be assured that you'll never be stuck drinking the same juices again and again.

Remember, the desire to lose weight begins and ends with you, but a juice cleanse may help you take the first steps toward lasting results.

Part One

JUICE CLEANSE BASICS

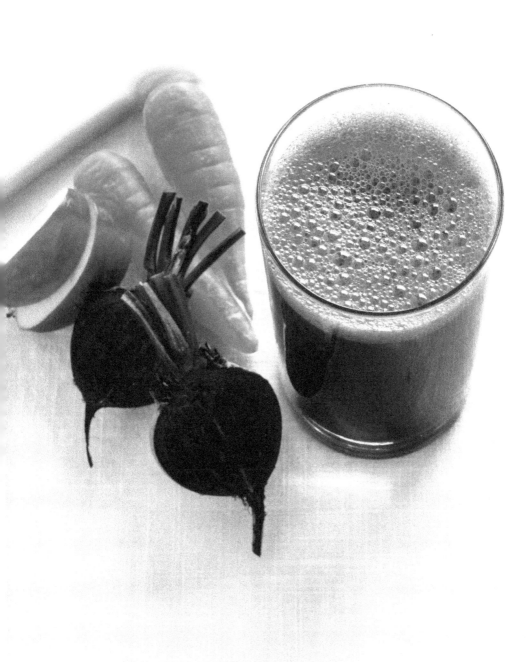

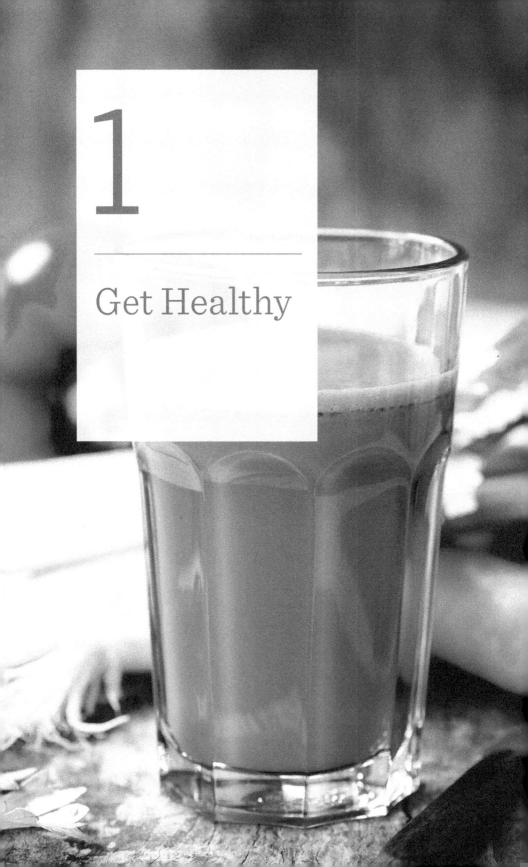

1

Get Healthy

Juicing is one of the fastest and most efficient ways to get the nutrients your body needs. Drinking a variety of fresh juices can help you feel better, look better, and have more energy.
—Bella NutriPro, "Benefits of Juicing"

Approximately 65 percent of Americans struggle with their weight. Most have tried a diet, or several, but gave up before reaching their goal. Even if the dieters reached their goal weight, they often quickly regained lost pounds once the diet ended.

Why is it so difficult to lose weight and keep it off? It all comes down to one simple reason: Most people are unwilling to change their habits.

If you want to lose weight, you have to change the way you eat.

Most Americans eat too much of the wrong foods—saturated fats, refined carbohydrates, and high-calorie and high-fat processed foods—and not enough fruits and vegetables. The average American eats fewer than half of the daily recommended amounts of fruits and vegetables, even though decades of research have shown that a largely or entirely plant-based diet is key to long-term health, and yes, lasting weight loss.

How do you break the cycle of junk eating and lose weight?

Drink your fruits and vegetables.

A short-term juice cleanse—over one, three, five, or seven days— is the easiest and most effective way to ensure you get the fruits and vegetables you need, and begin feeding your body the nutrients required to stimulate weight loss and ensure you keep the weight off.

WHAT IS A JUICE CLEANSE?

A juice cleanse means you limit your diet to only fresh vegetable and fruit juices and water; in this book, the juice cleanses are designed for one, three, five, or seven days. During a juice cleanse, you consume juice at every meal—breakfast, lunch, dinner, and even at snack time. The cleanse focuses on freshly made, unpasteurized juices made from a juicer. No processed, pasteurized juices found in stores are used, just fresh vegetables and fresh fruits with some herbs and spices to enhance flavors and provide variety.

Many companies now offer premade juices for cleansing, but these may include extra ingredients not necessarily desired or needed. Most of them contain far too many calories for short-term weight loss. By making the juices yourself, you control what's in them and make adjustments as necessary to fit your specific nutritional and caloric needs.

Juicing versus Smoothies

Don't confuse juicing with smoothies. They are quite different, especially when it comes to weight loss.

Juicing uses a machine that extracts water from produce while eliminating most, if not all, of its fiber. A lack of fiber means your digestive system doesn't have to work as hard to break down and absorb the nutrients in food.

Smoothies are fruits and vegetables pureed in a blender into a thick creamy texture, and the fiber is retained. Smoothies may include additional ingredients not approved for a juice cleanse, such as nut milk, yogurt, and sometimes protein powders.

While both may be effective weight-loss tools, juices usually have fewer calories than smoothies, because you drink just the juice from fruits and vegetables with no additives. With smoothies, your calories vary depending on the individual ingredients. Depending on the recipes, some smoothies may have as many calories as a full meal.

BENEFITS OF A JUICE CLEANSE

A short-term juice cleanse may propel you into a healthier lifestyle. And your changed eating habits may accelerate weight loss. The following is a list of some of the main benefits of juicing.

* *Appetite reduction.* Juicing may help eliminate the habit of "comfort eating"—the psychological connection you may have between eating and pleasure, and one of the main reasons people struggle with weight issues. When you no longer associate a certain food with happiness or contentment, you may begin to break that cycle and change your relationship with food for the better.

* *Elimination of questionable foods.* During a juice cleanse, all caffeine, alcohol, dairy, wheat, gluten, and fermented foods are restricted from your diet. Many people ignorantly suffer from a food allergy or intolerance to these common foods. Since a juice cleanse cuts out these common trigger foods for a specific period, you may notice you do not suffer from the same bloating, fatigue, or constipation as you did when you were eating pasta or drinking milk. When you resume eating whole foods, you will be able to identify potential problem foods.

* *Improved bone strength.* Two of the most essential nutrients for bone health and growth are calcium and magnesium. These two nutrients are found in abundance in a variety of green veg-

etables such as kale, broccoli, and collard greens. Including these vegetables in your fresh juice helps you build and maintain strong bones.

* *Improved eating habits.* People who battle weight issues are often caught in a cycle of poor eating, consuming too many high-calorie and processed foods, which contain too much saturated fat, sodium, and sugar. To compound the adverse effects of poor dietary choices, many of us overindulge during meals and eat portions that are much too large. A juice cleanse teaches more mindful eating habits and a better understanding of portion control.

* *Improved sleep habits.* Fresh juice helps improve sleep habits in two ways. First, leafy greens and other green vegetables contain high levels of magnesium, which helps you relax and mellow, preparing your body for sleep. Second, vitamin C, found in many fruits and vegetables, helps reduce stress reactions so you can avoid those late-night worry sessions.

* *Increased consumption of fruits and vegetables.* The recommended daily intake of fruits and vegetables is five to thirteen servings a day, or about $2\frac{1}{2}$ to $6\frac{1}{2}$ cups per day, depending on a person's caloric intake. As the Harvard School of Public Health calculates, the average person requires 2,000 calories a day to maintain ideal weight and health, so the estimated number of servings of fruits and vegetables per day is nine, or $4\frac{1}{2}$ cups. Most people don't come close to this on a regular basis. A juice cleanse dramatically increases your intake of these nutritional powerhouses.

* *Increased energy levels.* Drinking fresh juice can help increase your energy levels in a variety of ways. Most important, replacing unhealthful foods with raw juice can help cleanse your

body of the accumulated toxins that may be making you sluggish. Leafy greens and other vegetables also contain vitamins, which give your body a natural energy boost. When you begin to make positive changes to your health, you will feel more upbeat, happier, and confident, all of which are essential to lasting weight loss and weight maintenance.

- *Increased intake of natural probiotics.* Commercially produced and bottled juices are often pasteurized to increase their shelf life. This process, while ensuring that your bottle of orange juice lasts a week or two in the fridge, also kills off valuable enzymes and natural probiotics. Fresh juice, because it is not pasteurized, still contains these healthful elements.

- *Increased intake of nutrients.* The more fruits and vegetables you consume, the more vitamins, minerals, enzymes, and phytonutrients your body absorbs to maintain optimal health and promote weight loss. While cooking fruits and vegetables may destroy many of their nutrients, juices are made from raw ingredients that retain their nutrients. Up to 95 percent of vitamins and enzymes can be found in raw fruit and vegetable juice. According to the website Living Greens, a 16-ounce glass of raw juice has approximately the same nutrient content as 12 apples, 8 pounds of spinach, or 2 pounds of carrots. As an added bonus, by extracting the juice from the fiber, your body can more quickly and easily absorb the nutrients.

- *Increased longevity.* A study conducted by the Minerva Foundation Institute for Medical Research revealed that the nutrients found in raw juice help increase longevity. In addition to providing valuable vitamins and minerals, raw juice contains a nutrient called resveratrol, which helps prevent premature cell death.

- *Maximum detoxification.* To optimally support the body's natural detoxification organs—kidneys, liver, and digestive system—you need a broad range of plant-supplied nutrients with antioxidants and anti-inflammatories. Juicing super-nutrient-dense food allows the body to absorb more necessary nutrients to support the body's natural detox system.

- *Prevention of chronic diseases.* A healthful diet high in fiber, vitamins, and minerals has been shown to help stave off a number of chronic diseases, including diabetes, heart disease, and cancer. Vitamins and nutrients are abundantly available in raw juice.

- *Reduction of inflammation.* Fresh fruits and vegetables contain high levels of antioxidants, which perform a number of essential roles in the body, one of which is to reduce inflammation. Diets rich in acidic, fatty, and processed foods can cause inflammation and lead to other problems like heart disease and diabetes. The antioxidants found in fresh fruits and vegetables help reduce inflammation and prevent future health problems.

- *Rehydration of your body.* Your body demands water. Unfortunately, the average person drinks far less than he or she should. The Institute of Medicine suggests men should drink roughly 3 liters (about 100 ounces) of fluids a day, and women should drink around 2 liters (about 70 ounces). Any type of liquid counts toward this mark, according to the Mayo Clinic, and juicing can certainly provide your body with the liquids it needs to better run your detoxing machine. Some of the vegetables with the highest water content include celery, cucumber, and romaine lettuce.

TEN TIPS FOR GREAT JUICES

One of the best things about juicing is that you have the option to be as creative as you like. While many people prefer to follow recipes, you can create tasty masterpieces by just throwing together some of your favorite ingredients. To get the most out of your juicing and to speed your weight loss, follow these ten tips:

1. Include every color of the rainbow in your juices. Red ingredients tend to contain lycopene and manganese; green ingredients are rich in B vitamins, calcium, and beta-carotene.

2. Don't go overboard with fruit. Use half an apple or pear to sweeten green juices, but primarily use vegetables when juicing for weight loss.

3. Use a variety of ingredients to get the most out of your juices. Remember that less is more when it comes to juicing. You may need only one leaf of lettuce as part of a recipe, not several cups.

4. Stop by your local farmers' market or grocery store's organic section for deals on in-season produce. Not only will you save money, but you might also get to try something new.

5. If you are using a soft fruit or vegetable such as pineapple, juice that ingredient last. Soft ingredients may block the filter in your juicer, decreasing its efficacy for juicing other ingredients in the same batch.

6. Include a handful of fresh parsley in your juice for a burst of flavor and a quick energy boost.

7. After running your fruits and vegetables through the juicer, run the pulp through a second time. You might be surprised how much extra juice you get out of it.

8. Feel free to stir some powdered wheatgrass or dried spices into your juice to increase the flavor and the nutrient profile.

9. Use low-calorie vegetables like cucumbers and celery as the base for your juices. The water content in these veggies is high, and they have light, refreshing flavors.

10. If you must store your juice, place it in a glass container and remove as much air as possible before sealing and refrigerating it. Consume fresh juice within twenty-four hours.

WHAT TO EXPECT DURING A JUICE CLEANSE

Some people experience physical side effects during a juice cleanse. These vary from person to person and usually subside as your body adjusts. Keep in mind that these are only temporary and should pass with a minimum of discomfort. Furthermore, they are signs your body is cleansing well. Of course, if you find the symptoms too severe or uncomfortable, stop the cleanse. Here are some of the most common symptoms you may encounter:

- *Aches and pains.* Withdrawal symptoms from salt, sugar, or caffeine may cause some headaches or stomachaches. Some people, however, notice their arthritis and other pains lessen or even disappear.

- *Bloating.* You might feel bloated at times, but this is normal. Drinking fresh juices flushes out your intestines and gets rid of fecal matter. During this time, microorganisms inside you are releasing gas, which is why you may feel bloated. A cup of chamomile tea may help relieve bloating.

- *Bowel movements.* Loose bowel movements sometimes occur, since vegetables and fruits can have a natural laxative effect. This process is helping eliminate toxins and clean out your digestive system. Make sure to drink plenty of water and stay well hydrated.

- *Hunger pangs.* Hunger pangs occur most often during the first and second days of a cleanse. This is to be expected since you are making sudden changes to your eating habits. You may be surprised how quickly they subside once you get into the rhythm of a juice cleanse.

- *Weakness.* Your stamina may be lower than normal. A lack of energy may make you feel cold, because your body is not burning fuel to stay warm. You may also feel sleepy, so make sure you stick to your regular sleep schedule and take naps when needed.

TOP TEN JUICING QUESTIONS

1. *Am I just losing water weight?*

Most of your initial weight loss may be attributed to water weight, but whether you lose water or fat from a juice cleanse depends on how much you weighed before the cleanse. If you are twenty or more pounds overweight, your body may begin to tap into its fat stores, since you will be consuming fewer calories than usual. A juice cleanse is meant to get you started on your weight-loss goals. Use whatever success you achieve on the scale as a sign that you are heading in a new and healthier direction.

2. *How often should I cleanse?*

A juice cleanse should not be adopted as an ongoing diet plan. After you have completed the juice cleanse, you may feel the need to revisit a cleanse now and again for short periods to reenergize your ongoing weight management if you have slipped into your previous bad eating habits and/or have begun to gain weight. You may also repeat a cleanse when you feel especially fatigued, have trouble sleeping, or need to recharge yourself.

3. *Is juice healthier than whole fruits and vegetables?*

While juices hydrate and supply nutrients to the body, there's no reliable scientific research to support claims that juicing your produce is healthier than eating it whole. But if your goal is to increase your intake of fruits and vegetables, drinking juice instead of eating a plate of produce is easier for many people.

4. *Should I exercise during a juice cleanse?*
Your daily calorie intake during a cleanse will be lower than usual. Since your body needs a certain number of calories to function on a daily basis, juicing may not provide the necessary calories to support a regular exercise routine or the nutrients needed for healing and recovery. Registered dietitian Cynthia Sass says that while following a limited eating plan like a juice cleanse, exercising may create unwanted side effects, such as fatigue, dizziness, and nausea. So give your body time off during your cleanse.

5. *Will I notice any significant change in my bowel movement?*
Each person's digestive system is unique, but many people will experience a slight increase in elimination frequency and a softer bowel movement than usual. A juice cleanse helps your body purge itself of waste and toxins, so there might be a sight change in color and consistency of your stool. If you have any health concerns, please see your health care provider for advice.

6. *Will I become more tempted to binge eat?*
Binge eating occurs when you become so hungry that you consume large amounts of food in a short period of time. You will encounter episodes of hunger where you will be tempted to break down and eat a lot of whole foods. The reason is that in tandem with a reduced calorie intake, you also may miss the satisfaction of chewing food. This temptation to eat is normal, but the juices for all meals and snacks in this book will help curb cravings and prevent the urge to binge eat.

7. *Will I get headaches?*

Headaches, which may occur during the first few days, are usually caused by sudden withdrawal from caffeine and sugar. This is why it is recommended to begin eliminating foods and drinks that contain caffeine and sugar several days before you begin your cleanse. The headaches will pass. In the meantime, taking a relaxing hot bath or an afternoon nap, or drinking green tea—1 cup has about 70 percent less caffeine than coffee—may help. Avoid taking aspirin or ibuprofen unless the headaches become too severe or distracting.

8. *Who should not do a juice cleanse?*

A juice cleanse is not recommended for people undergoing chemotherapy, people with diabetes, those with nutritional deficiencies, and individuals with kidney disease. Pregnant and nursing women as well as children should not do a juice cleanse. Some of the vitamins and nutrients in juices may interfere with certain medications; if you have a current medical condition or are taking daily medications, check with your physician before following a juice cleanse.

9. *Is juicing expensive?*

Quality juicers range in price from $100 to $300, depending on the specific features, which is a small price to pay considering how often you will use it—during the cleanse and afterward. Buying a juicer is the only upfront cost for following a juice cleanse. Since your grocery store purchases will consist mainly of fresh produce, you will eliminate higher-priced items like meat, processed foods, and dairy products, so you may even experience a savings in your food bills.

10. *Can I work while doing a juice cleanse?*

Yes, but keep in mind that your energy levels will be lower than normal. If you have a physical job or one that requires high levels of concentration for safety, it is recommended you do a juice cleanse during vacation time or over a long weekend. Also, doing your cleanse while at home offers a more comfortable and stress-free environment to help you through the initial adjustments while you cope with possible side effects. If you feel tired or have a headache, it is often better to be at home than at the office.

2

Lose Weight

It is important to keep in mind the role of a juice cleanse in overall weight loss, and understand its limitations. It is not a magic meal plan that will create dramatic results in a short time. Nor will it suddenly "cure" any existing ailments.

A short-duration juice cleanse—one day, three days, five days, or seven days—may instill many positive changes that may initiate weight loss and create a solid foundation for you to follow. Use a short-term juice cleanse to do the following:

- ◆ *Break bad habits that contribute to weight gain.* If you're substantially overweight, then you probably have poor eating habits, such as frequently indulging your sweet tooth with ice cream or having a couple of glasses of wine every evening. Whatever the causes, the first step to long-term weight loss is to break those bad habits. Often, adopting a simple, well-defined, and structured meal plan like a juice cleanse is the best way to eliminate your previous eating habits by forcing yourself to forgo your usual choices.

- ◆ *Create new and healthier eating habits proven to be successful for long-term weight loss.* Most people overeat because their portions are too large. We either super-size everything or feel compelled to fill large bowls and plates to the rim. To stimulate weight loss and keep it off, gain better control of your portion sizes and consume only what you need and nothing more. A juice cleanse, with its fixed portions, may be helpful in teaching you how to control portions.

* *Improve your natural detox system through an increased intake of essential vitamins, minerals, and phytochemicals that are linked to long-term weight loss.* Your body already possesses the best detoxification system possible. The liver, kidneys, and digestive system work constantly to filter out toxins and increase the absorption of vital vitamins, minerals, and nutrients. Increasing your intake of fruits and vegetables through a juice cleanse feeds your body's systems to ensure they can do their job.

A juice cleanse also gives your detox system a much-deserved respite to repair itself. Juices require less of the stomach's digestive processing (churning, acid, and pepsin) to extract nutrients compared with the digestion of foods high in saturated fats, refined carbs, and additives, so with juice, your body doesn't need to work as hard. When the stomach works less, so do the kidneys and liver, as there are fewer toxins to filter. The following is a closer look at your body's detox system and its vital role in weight management.

Kidneys

Your kidneys work around the clock to reduce fat storage. One of their main daily duties is to remove waste and excess fluids from your bloodstream. Every twenty-four hours, your kidneys process about 200 quarts of blood. During this time, the kidneys help remove about 2 quarts of waste, including extra water and potential fat-producing substances, such as food the body doesn't use. Because the kidneys work so hard with no rest, you have to keep them healthy so they can continue to do their job. Unhealthy kidneys mean less waste is moved out of your body and more fat is stored.

How do your kidneys get overworked? Too much protein is usually to blame. Some estimates suggest the average sedentary American eats about 50 percent more protein than the daily recommended 40 to 80 grams. For example, a woman whose ideal weight is 130 pounds needs only about 48 to 60 grams of protein per day or 4 ounces of meat and 16 ounces of milk; a man weighing 175 pounds requires 64 to 80 daily grams of protein per day or 6 ounces of meat and 16 ounces of milk.

Protein isn't all bad, of course; yet, too much of anything can have a negative effect, and protein is no exception. Kidneys have to strain to filter excess protein. Consuming more than necessary makes it tougher to excrete waste and toxins, and thus prevent stored fat.

A juice cleanse helps the kidneys is several ways. First, since it reduces or eliminates your normal protein consumption, you give your kidneys a well-deserved break. It also increases your intake of vitamins D_3 and K, which have been shown to support and strengthen your kidneys. In 2013, the *American Journal of Kidney Diseases* published findings of a close association between vitamin D levels and chronic kidney disease. In fact, new research from the *American Journal of Kidney Diseases* found that people who are deficient in vitamin D are more than twice as likely to demonstrate signs of potential kidney disease. The current recommended daily allowance for vitamin D is 600 IUs. Yet the average person's intake of vitamin D from food is fewer than 300 IUs, according to the 2005–2006 National Health and Nutrition Examination Survey.

Finally, well-hydrated kidneys are healthy kidneys. Dehydration strains your kidneys because it lowers your blood pressure and disrupts autoregulated blood flow to them. That may eventually lead to kidney damage. The color of your urine can guide your hydration level; it should be straw to lemonade color. A juice cleanse helps meet your body's hydration needs by increasing your fluid intake.

Digestion

Your digestive system—intestines and stomach—plays two key roles in weight loss and weight management: absorption and digestion. Your stomach breaks down and digests nutrients you eat to fuel your body, and your intestines are the gatekeeper; they allow the nutritionally sound material in through absorption, and get rid of the bad stuff such as viruses and heavy metals like arsenic, lead, and cadmium.

One class of nutrient that goes a long way to supporting your digestive system is flavonoids. They are compounds typically found in most fruits and vegetables as well as in green and black tea. As an antioxidant, flavonoids work as an anti-inflammatory nutrient. Inflammation of the digestive tract inhibits the absorption of good nutrients, so keeping your stomach and intestine lining healthy and blood flowing smoothly helps nutrients get absorbed and transferred to other parts of your body. A juice cleanse cuts out solid foods for a short time and gives your stomach and intestines an opportunity to rest and return to an optimal state.

Liver

The liver stores all the toxins that your body cannot break down, including excess fat. A healthy liver contains some fat, but it's important not to add to it. If your liver's total weight climbs above 10 percent fat, you can suffer from fatty liver. When this happens, extra fat builds up in the liver cells, which slows liver function and makes you feel fatigued. When the liver can't fully metabolize fats circulating in the blood, it begins to store them.

What causes fatty liver? Extreme and even moderate weight gain is the main culprit, but so is a heavy-food diet. You can cleanse a fatty liver by eliminating high-fat foods or foods that contain saturated fat—and no doubt have led to your current weight gain—and increasing your intake of plant sterols and stanols and vitamins B_6, B_{12}, and E.

- *Plant sterols and stanols.* Sterols and stanols are fats found in all plant foods. They block the absorption of cholesterol in the small intestine, which may lower LDL (bad) cholesterol without affecting HDL (good) cholesterol. Lowering LDL cholesterol and keeping overall cholesterol levels in check may help the liver be more effective at filtering toxins and stop fatty buildup in the body that may translate to weight gain.

- *Vitamins B_6 and B_{12}*: Vitamin B_6 improves liver metabolism essentially by keeping its engine revved up. Vitamin B_6 assists in turning carbohydrates in the liver into energy, which helps the liver more effectively move out toxins and balance hormones. It also assists the liver in breaking down fat, and fatty liver is often associated with a vitamin B_{12} deficiency. According to Dr. Christine Gerbstadt, studies have shown that patients with fatty liver disease improved their condition when taking recommended amounts of B_{12}.

- *Vitamin E*: A fat-soluble vitamin with antioxidant properties, vitamin E also helps improve liver function in people who suffer from advanced fatty liver. In fact, a study published in the *New England Journal of Medicine* found that among a group of almost 250 people, 43 percent improved their liver function after taking vitamin E (800 IUs) compared with only 19 percent in the placebo group.

HOW JUICING CAN HELP YOU LOSE WEIGHT

Simply adding fresh juice to your daily diet is not a guaranteed way to lose weight. In fact, it might have the opposite effect. If you have been trying to lose weight, you already know the importance of burning more calories than you take in on a daily basis. It should go without saying that adding extra calories to your daily intake will not help you lose weight. When you're not replacing your entire day's meal with juices during a juice cleanse, incorporate juicing into your dietary routine as a replacement for high-calorie snacks, or even a meal or two. By using fresh juice to replace high-calorie foods, you can bring your daily calorie count down and improve your weight-loss efforts.

Use the chart to estimate your daily calorie needs based on your age, sex, and activity level. Keep in mind that these numbers are for weight maintenance.

Now that you know what the calorie range is for you to maintain your current weight, you can begin to think about reducing that number to lose weight. One pound of fat is equal to about 3,500 calories. Thus in order to lose one pound per week, you should plan to eliminate this many calories from your weekly intake. This averages to about 500 calories per day. Studies have shown, however, that weight lost over a longer period of time is easier to sustain. Consider reducing your daily calorie count by only 300 calories per day. This is where juicing comes in—after you give your body a reset with a full juice cleanse, you can continue to use juices for quick and easy low-calorie meals that are also high in nutrients.

WHY A JUICE CLEANSE FOR WEIGHT LOSS WORKS

Lasting weight loss does not happen overnight or over a long weekend. To drop those extra pounds, and keep them off, you need to adopt new eating habits. A juice cleanse is not a miracle program, but it is based on actual nutritional research. In fact, a study from the *American Journal of Clinical Nutrition* found that consuming more produce was the key to long-term weight loss. Researchers at the University of Pittsburgh Department of Health and Physical Activity concluded that eating more fruits and vegetables and less

Estimated Calorie Needs per Day

Source: USDA, Estimated Energy Requirements (EER)

	MALE				FEMALE		
Age	Sedentary	Moderately Active	Active	Age	Sedentary	Moderately Active	Active
18	2,400	2,800	3,200	18	2,400	2,800	3,200
19–20	2,600	2,800	3,000	19–20	2,600	2,800	3,000
21–25	2,400	2,800	3,000	21–25	2,400	2,800	3,000
26–30	2,400	2,600	3,000	26–30	2,400	2,600	3,000
31–35	2,400	2,600	3,000	31–35	2,400	2,600	3,000
36–40	2,400	2,600	2,800	36–40	2,400	2,600	2,800
41–45	2,200	2,600	2,800	41–45	2,200	2,600	2,800
46–50	2,200	2,400	2,800	46–50	2,200	2,400	2,800
51–55	2,200	2,400	2,800	51–55	2,200	2,400	2,800
56–60	2,200	2,400	2,600	56–60	2,200	2,400	2,600
61–65	2,000	2,400	2,600	61–65	2,000	2,400	2,600
66–70	2,000	2,200	2,600	66–70	2,000	2,200	2,600
71–75	2,000	2,200	2,600	71–75	2,000	2,200	2,600
76+	2,000	2,200	2,400	76+	2,000	2,200	2,400

meat and cheese was an important predictor for long-term weight loss, especially for postmenopausal women who may have more trouble losing weight. A juice cleanse is directly in line with these studies.

Juicing also helps teach you to control your eating. If your weight gain is the result of overindulging and consuming too many high-calorie meals, a juice cleanse may reverse that pattern. During a cleanse you are introduced to low-calorie meals, and because you drink instead of eat, you learn about portion control. According to a study in the *American Journal of Preventive Medicine*, low-calorie meals and portion control are the two leading factors of long-term weight-loss management.

Finally, juicing introduces the role of snacking into your daily diet, which is a powerful tool for curbing appetite and reaching weight-loss goals. In fact, according to the website ScienceDaily, researchers found that women dieters who had either a food or drink midmorning snack lost an average of 7 percent of their total body weight. The experts noted that the best snacks for successful weight loss should have no more than 200 calories and include non-starchy vegetables and fresh fruits—all of which are central to a juice cleanse.

ESSENTIAL NUTRIENTS FOR WEIGHT LOSS

If weight loss is your goal, you shouldn't have to sacrifice your health to achieve it. While incorporating juicing into your dietary routine is a great way to encourage weight loss, there are a few key things you should be aware of before you start. The trick to losing weight while juicing is to take in fewer calories than you expend, but it is still important to fuel your body with the nutrients it needs within that lower calorie count. Fortunately, fresh juices are rich in nutrients, including antioxidants, vitamins, minerals, and more.

B Vitamins

Vitamins B_1, B_2, B_5, and B_6 are essential for energy conversion from food. B vitamins help activate crucial enzymes in the process of the absorption of carbs, fats, and proteins. Without B vitamins calories are often stored as fat instead of burned. B vitamins also boost the metabolism and help curb cravings. Good sources are spinach, banana, sweet potato, beet greens, and asparagus.

28

Calcium

The average adult requires about 1,000 mg of calcium per day. Calcium not only helps maintain bone health and density, but it also helps regulate blood pressure. The best vegetable sources for calcium include collard greens, kale, bok choy, mustard greens, and broccoli.

Chromium

Chromium is essential for increasing the body's sensitivity to insulin. Increased insulin sensitivity helps support weight loss because without this mineral, blood sugar levels in the body can be elevated, creating cravings. Great sources of chromium are sweet potato, broccoli, corn, ginger, cinnamon, and cumin.

Iron

Iron is an essential mineral for the body. It helps your red blood cells carry oxygen throughout the body to vital organs. If your iron stores get too low, you may end up feeling tired and sluggish—less inclined to exercise and to maintain your diet. Some of the best iron-packed foods to include in juicing are spinach, parsley, coconut, and Swiss chard. Vitamin C is another important nutrient because it helps increase the ability of your red blood cells to carry oxygen. Some natural sources of vitamin C include oranges, red bell peppers, kiwi, grapefruit, Brussels sprouts, and cantaloupe.

Magnesium

This mineral is crucial for almost every function that occurs in your body. It can be very beneficial when trying to lose weight because it boosts the metabolism, promotes a healthy digestive system, and can help reduce the cravings you might have for sweet foods. Magnesium is found in spinach, Swiss chard, beet greens, turnip greens, and summer squash.

Protein

This macronutrient is essential for building the muscles, tissues, and nerves in the body, and it is also an important fuel source. If you do not consume enough protein, your body will take it from your muscles. While this may not seem like a big deal, you should be aware that muscle burns more calories than fat, so you are better off keeping what muscle you have. Including vegetables like green peas, spinach, broccoli, and alfalfa sprouts in your juice can help increase your protein intake during a cleanse.

EXERCISE RECOMMENDATIONS

In order to jump-start and maintain weight loss while juicing, you should plan to incorporate moderate exercise into your weekly routine. Many studies recommend thirty minutes of moderate exercise—such as walking or hiking—three times per week for good health. This is a good starting point, but the more exercise you get, the more calories you burn and the more quickly weight comes off. A simple way to get in daily exercise is to take a quick fifteen-minute walk during your lunch break and when you get home from work. You can also work some extra activity into your day by taking the stairs instead of the elevator, by parking farther from the front entrance, and by doing simple stretches and exercises while cooking or relaxing at home each day.

While increasing your daily exercise is a great way to lose weight, you should be cautious about becoming too active during your juice cleanse. While a cleanse helps spur weight loss, you could experience detrimental side effects if you try to engage in vigorous exercise while on a cleanse. Strenuous activities like strength training or running are not recommended while engaging in a low-calorie diet, so be very careful. As always, it is a good idea to drink plenty of water to stay hydrated while you exercise.

Although it is safe to exercise while juicing, especially when trying to lose weight, it is important to listen to your body, as well. If you are already active and follow a daily exercise routine, then continue it at the same intensity as long as you have the energy. The first couple days of your cleanse might produce fatigue, so wait until you feel good again to continue your routine. Don't overdo exercise by adding new components to the workout or miles of distance to your run. Your body will not have many extra calories to support extra exercise. Working out too hard without enough fuel can create uncomfortable side effects such as lowered metabolic rate, nausea, headaches, dizziness, and fatigue. Your muscle mass could suffer, as well, which increases your risk of injury.

The key to exercising while doing a juice cleanse is to focus on light to moderate exercise, because this type of exercise enhances and stimulates the systems in the body that help the elimination process. These systems include the lymphatic system, perspiration, and digestion. The lymphatic system is particularly important when cleansing because it carries most of the waste in the body to the elimination organs while producing antibodies and white blood cells. Stimulating the lymphatic system will enhance your cleanse experience and support weight-loss goals.

Some important points to consider when exercising during your juice cleanse are:

* Do not try to build muscle; the calorie intake during your juice cleanse will not provide your body the support it needs to

increase bulk. You can lift lighter weights or do moderate circuit training, but save the power lifting until you are finished with your juice cleanse.

* Try less impactful and strenuous exercise, such as yoga, which can stretch your body, clear your mind, and enhance your breathing. Take a few beginner classes at your local gym or find a dedicated studio to give this ancient exercise form a try. You might find yourself continuing yoga after your juice cleanse is over and you reach your weight goal.

* Continue your favorite familiar exercise routine but reduce the intensity by about half in deference to your reduced calorie intake. Never attempt to do a weight-loss juice cleanse or any juice cleanse when training for an athletic event. You will find that your physical need for carbohydrates, protein, and even fat will not be met and your performance will suffer.

* Try swimming for exercise. Swimming is a wonderful choice because it puts very little stress on joints due to the weight-lessness of the water. Whenever possible swim in fresh water or pools that use salt to clean their water instead of chlorine. Juice cleanses detox the body, and even if weight loss is the goal, exposing yourself to chemicals is not compatible to that process.

* Take a break for the first few days of your juice cleanse so your body can get used to the effects and process. Work your way back up to a normal or slightly reduced exercise routine if you are doing a five- or seven-day cleanse.

* If you want to be very active and feel hungry, add an extra juice to your day. Going into a severe calorie deficit because you are burning a great deal of calories can be extremely damaging. It can also completely sabotage any weight-loss success you

might have achieved and wreck your metabolism. Listen to your body. If necessary, stop your juice cleanse. The goal is to enhance your body's health; only you know your limits.

EXERCISE LOG

The best chance of launching a successful exercise routine is to keep track of exactly when and what you do during the week. This type of journal will also allow you to increase reps, weight, duration, and type of exercise using the previous week as a guideline. Use this journal after you complete your cleanse and have established new, healthful eating habits. You've already done half the work, so keep up your weight loss (or weight maintenance) with regular exercise.

WEEK:

DAY OF THE WEEK	EXERCISE	DURATION/WEIGHT
Monday		
Tuesday		
Wednesday		
Thursday		
Friday		
Saturday		
Sunday		

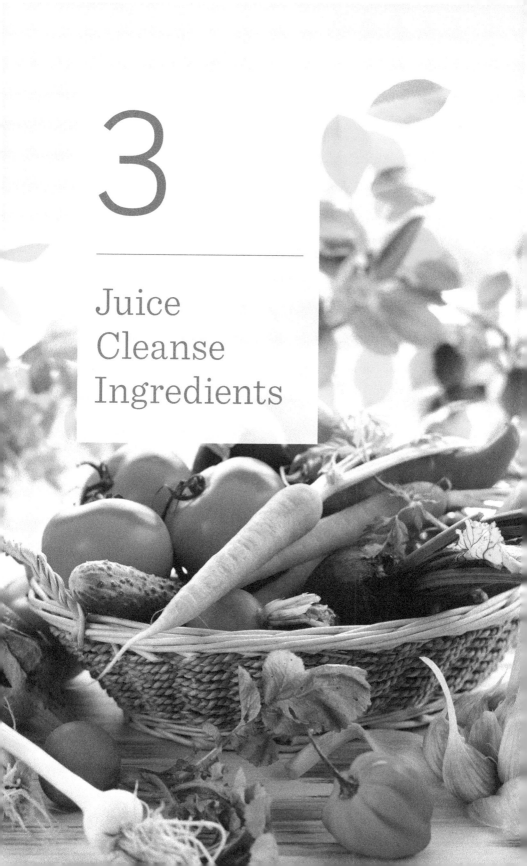

3

Juice Cleanse Ingredients

Detoxification is what your body does naturally to neutralize, transform, or get rid of unwanted materials or toxins. It is a primary function of the body, constantly working and interacting with all other functions of the body. . . . [Detoxification] is about improving and optimizing the function of your body's own detoxification systems.
—Frank Lipman, MD, "What Do You Mean by Detox?"

The success of juicing for weight loss lies in your selection of fruits and vegetables. With so many choices, you can create an almost unlimited variety of juices. Before you head to the produce section, you first need to understand how to choose the best produce for your cleanse. You want to ensure that you juice only the highest-quality produce to obtain nutritional benefits. Many herbs and spices have their own unique weight-loss properties and may be added to juices to enhance flavor. Here, you will learn why you should use only fresh, raw fruits and vegetables in your juice cleanse along with herbs and spices. You'll also learn how to prepare your juices.

WHY MAKE JUICES FROM SCRATCH?

When it comes to juice, fresh is always best. By making your own juices, you have control over when it was made and can ensure that no additives or preservatives dilute the juice's nutritional quality.

Canned, bottled, or boxed fruit and vegetable juices found on the grocery shelf are automatically inferior to fresh juice for a variety of reasons. Since they have to last longer and not spoil, premade juices are exposed to a pasteurization process to kill microorganisms. This involves heating the beverage to a temperature of 250°F—a process that destroys most of a juice's natural enzymes, vitamins, and minerals. Also, many brands add preservatives, artificial colors, and refined sugars that even further deplete a juice's nutritional values. Don't be fooled by labels that promise "100 percent juice" or "all natural" juice. These marketing ploys do not tell the real story of how the juice was made.

To ensure you get only the purest and healthiest juices with no additives, you need to make them yourself with only the freshest produce—organic, too, if possible. This way your juices are always packed with the vital nutrients you need for your cleanse.

INGREDIENTS TO INCLUDE AND EXCLUDE

The amazing thing about juicers is that they can reduce even the toughest vegetables and fruits to flavorful juice. However, there are some things that simply do not juice well.

If weight loss is your goal, be careful about using ingredients that have a high sugar or starch content. Not only are these ingredients higher in calories but they may not be as rich as other ingredients in certain vitamins and minerals.

FRUITS VERSUS VEGETABLES

Before you begin your juice cleanse, you need to understand how fruit and vegetables will fit into the meal plan, and how to select the best ones.

The juices you make for your cleanse will be approximately three parts vegetables to one part fruit—or 80 to 90 percent vegetables to 10 to 20 percent fruit. There are some exceptions, but this ratio ensures that you will limit how much fructose, or natural fruit sugar, you eat. When you consume whole fruit, and its fiber,

Some foods that don't juice well:

Apple seeds
Avocados (too soft)
Bananas (too soft)
Citrus peels, except lemons
    and limes (not toxic, just
    hard to digest)
Dried fruit
Nuts and seeds
Papaya peels (may damage
juicer, not edible)

Some foods to limit in your weight-loss juices:

Berries
Mangos
Oranges
Pineapple
Sweet potatoes
Taro root

Some of the best foods to include for weight loss:

Apples
Arugula
Beets
Bell peppers
Broccoli
Cabbage
Carrots
Celery
Collard greens
Cranberries
Cucumbers
Fennel
Fresh herbs
Ginger
Kale
Lemons
Limes
Radishes
Romaine lettuce
Spinach
Tomatoes
Turnips
Watercress
Wheatgrass

fructose is absorbed slowly. But when the fiber is removed through juicing, the fructose hits the bloodstream quicker, which may result in sugar spikes (bursts of energy) and sugar crashes (sudden drops in energy). You can avoid this by using fewer fruits and more vegetables in your juices.

Many of the foods used in juicing, such as most fruits and nonstarchy vegetables, are low glycemic. The glycemic index (GI) ranks carbohydrates on a scale of 0 to 100 based on how they raise blood sugar levels. Low GI foods with a score of 55 or less are more slowly digested, which keeps you feeling full for longer and delays cravings and hunger pangs.

Whenever possible, you should juice only organic fruits and vegetables. This advice might be tempting to ignore, as organic produce may be more expensive and sometimes may not be as readily available as conventional produce. But the point of a juice cleanse is to eliminate toxins and support your natural detox system, and thus help stimulate weight loss. Using fruits and vegetables that may contain chemicals, toxins, or other contaminations can defeat the purpose of the cleanse.

Organic produce is grown without pesticides or fertilizers made with synthetic ingredients. According to the website for the Food and Drug Administration (FDA), all organic produce carries the US Department of Agriculture (USDA) seal and is labeled as 100 percent organic. If you buy produce from a farmers' market, ask if the produce was grown organically, as they may not carry the USDA seal.

Even if you choose not to go the 100 percent organic route, you should at least buy the "dirty dozen" organic. The dirty dozen are fruits and vegetables the Environmental Working Group (EWG) has identified as being the most contaminated. The EWG has also identified what it calls the "clean fifteen" for nonorganic produce that has the least amount of contamination. If you're watching your food budget, the clean fifteen are the best options to buy nonorganic. See Appendix A for a list of the dirty dozen and clean fifteen produce.

TIPS FOR BUYING FRUITS AND VEGETABLES

Since your juice cleanse revolves around fruit and vegetables, you need to take care when shopping. Avoid impulse shopping and be selective: Purchase only the highest-quality produce to ensure you enjoy the most health benefits from your juice cleanse. Here are some basic tips from the Academy of Nutrition and Dietetics to follow when loading up for your cleanse:

* Purchase fresh produce that is not bruised or damaged. Fruits and vegetables that have been on the shelves for a long time will decay more quickly and lose their nutritional quality faster.

* Bag fresh fruits and vegetables to keep them segregated from potential bacteria from meat, poultry, and seafood products.

* Purchase fresh fruits and vegetables when they are in season to obtain fresher, more nutrient-rich produce typically at cheaper prices.

* Shop at farmers' markets whenever possible, where you can usually find locally grown, in-season produce, which is often fresher than produce that may have been shipped internationally to your supermarket.

* Use your fruits and vegetables within a week; the longer produce sits after being picked, the more nutrients it loses.

* Store fresh fruits and vegetables in a refrigerator set at 40°F. This helps keep your produce fresher longer.

Wax Coating on Fruits and Vegetables

Many vegetables and fruits grown in warmer climates, such as apples, pears, and cucumbers, make their own natural waxy coating to prevent too much moisture from being lost. Produce is sometimes cleaned of any dirt after being harvested, but this process may remove the natural wax. Therefore, waxes are applied to help maintain quality from farm to store, protecting produce from bruising and disease while giving the fruit and vegetables a clean, shiny look. Not much wax is used. In fact, most produce is covered with only a drop or two of wax. Produce shippers and supermarkets in the United States are required to label fresh fruits and vegetables that have been waxed. Look for signs that include wording such as: coated with food-grade vegetable-, petroleum-, beeswax-, or shellac-based wax or resin to maintain freshness.

Wax coatings are just a thin layer, but long-term health risks are unknown. Removing the skin is the only way to remove the wax. Use a peeler that takes off only a thin layer of skin. Many of the vitamins and minerals of fruits and vegetables lie right below the skin's surface, so you don't want to peel away the nutrients. The nonorganic fruits and vegetables that are often covered with wax include:

* Apples
* Bell peppers
* Cucumbers
* Eggplant
* Lemons and limes
* Oranges

FRUITS AND VEGETABLES FOR JUICING

Fruits and vegetables play an important role when it comes to effective weight loss. Many are rich sources of vitamin C, and a 2005 article in the *Journal of the American College of Nutrition* reported that people with adequate levels of vitamin C are able to oxidize 30 percent more fat during moderate exercise compared to those with lower vitamin C levels. Many fruits and vegetables also contain good amounts of vitamin A, which can help strengthen your immune system and fight off possible infection to keep you active and healthy; staying active is a necessary component of continued weight loss and weight management. Vitamin A also keeps your digestive system healthy and aids in better nutrient absorption.

Some of the best vegetables for stimulating weight loss are the cruciferous kind. They are low in calories; for instance, one cup of chopped broccoli contains just 31 calories. They also have a lower glycemic index, which means they don't cause spikes in your blood sugar that lead to the release of insulin—the hormone that converts calories to fat. Finally, for women, these vegetables may help improve estrogen levels, asserts Ori Hofmekler, author of *The Warrior Diet*. An imbalance in estrogen metabolism is often linked with a diet low in vegetables, and may cause your body to store more fat. Cruciferous vegetables contain a large amount of diindolylmethane, a compound that can restore the balance of estrogen metabolites.

Of course, there is an almost endless supply of fruits and vegetables you may juice as part of a cleanse. For a detailed breakdown of the nutrients in the fruits and vegetables that are the staples of weight-loss juices, see Appendix B.

Buying a Juicer

There are several types of juicers on the market, so make sure you get the best model for your juicing needs.

Centrifugal juicers. These are the most common type of juicers, especially for people on a budget or who are new to juicing. They shred produce with a sharp blade, then separate the pulp by spinning at high speed through a strainer screen to yield pulp-free juice. These machines can juice dense vegetables and fruits like carrots, beets, and apples but are less efficient at processing leafy greens. Wrap leafy greens such as kale or collards around more dense produce such as apples or carrots for successful centrifugal juicing. The centrifugal juicer's main downside, especially for raw food enthusiasts, is that the machine generates about two degrees Fahrenheit of heat, which may break down some of a juice's enzymes and nutrients. Another possible concern with this type of juicer is that oxygen is dissolved in the juice due to the high-speed spinning. This added oxygen decreases the shelf life of the finished juice, so you need to drink it right away.

Masticating or cold-press juicers (single gear/single auger). These juicers use an auger to crush the juice from foods, which creates a higher juice yield than a high-speed centrifugal juicer. They can handle any type of ingredient easily, even greens and herbs, which can clog centrifugal juicers. There is no heat produced during the juicing process in a masticating juicer, and the juice can be stored up to forty-eight hours in the fridge, which is perfect for people who want to do big batches. The two main downsides of masticating juicers are that they typically are more expensive and they have smaller feeder chutes, so ingredients need to be cut into smaller pieces before they can be juiced.

Triturating juicers. This is the most effective juicer you can buy. It is basically a masticating juicer that uses two gears or augers instead of one. The juiced ingredients are ground up very slowly between two rollers, producing the highest nutrient quality and juice yield. You can juice any ingredient in the triturating juicer with great results except some more fibrous products such as pineapple. This juicer produces no heat or oxygen-filled foam, and is quiet while running. The downsides of this juicer are that it is the most expensive type and you will need to cut your produce into small pieces to fit it through the feed chute, so it will take more time to create your juices.

Wheatgrass juicers. These juicers come in both manual and electric models. The wheatgrass juicer is specifically for wheatgrass as well as other greens and soft fruits such as grapes. If you don't plan on using a great deal of wheatgrass or have a masticating or triturating juicer, you will not need a wheatgrass juicer.

FRESH HERBS AND SPICES FOR JUICING

There are many fresh herbs and dried spices to add to your juices for extra flavor and health benefits beyond weight loss. Here are some healthful choices.

Fresh Herbs

* *Cilantro*

This leafy herb is used in Mexican, Middle Eastern, and Asian dishes. It also is a source of limonene, a food chemical that acts as a mild appetite suppressant and helps block fat buildup. Because cilantro is grown in sandy soil, wash the herb well in cold water. Both the leaves and stems may be used for juicing.

* *Dill*

Dill helps promote stronger digestion, which supports your natural detox system as well as a quicker digestion of fatty foods. It has a sweet, citrusy, and slightly bitter taste. Cut off the roots, wash it well, and use the leaves and stems in juicing.

* *Oregano*

Oregano is loaded with antioxidants that support your natural detox systems as well as help you fight unhealthful food temptations. Research from the Institute of Food Technologists found that everyday spices, including oregano, make vegetables more appetizing than high-calorie meals. The scientists noted that this effect may help people resist the temptation for unhealthful meals that contribute to weight gain. Use the leaves and discard the stems.

◆ *Parsley*

Parsley contains a high amount of chlorophyll and carotenes. The chlorophyll helps tone down the odor and taste of many spicy foods. It also has been used for treating urinary tract infections, kidney stones, various gastrointestinal disorders, osteoarthritis, and anemia among other conditions. Wash it well and use the stems and leaves when juicing.

◆ *Tarragon*

This long-leaved herb has a slightly peppery taste and contains an impressive amount of iron in a single teaspoon. It also has polyphenolic compounds, which help regulate blood sugar levels and control appetite. You can use either fresh leaves, stripped from their stems, or dried tarragon for juices; dried tarragon is easier to find and measure.

◆ *Thyme*

Thyme has a subtle, dry aroma with a slight minty flavor. It also aids in digestion and is often added to foods that may cause gastrointestinal problems. Strip the leaves from the stems for juicing.

Spices

◆ *Black Pepper*

A pinch or two of black pepper may be added to almost every juice recipe. It helps improve digestion by stimulating your taste buds and increasing hydrochloric acid secretion in your stomach, which is needed to break down proteins and other nutrients. Pepper also helps with weight loss as the peppercorn's outer layer stimulates the breakdown of fat cells. Use freshly ground peppercorns in a pepper mill, not preground pepper.

* *Cardamom*

An aromatic and sweet spice, cardamom is often used to improve digestion. It also contains small amounts of melatonin, which researchers at the University of Granada have found may help control weight gain. Add a pinch of ground cardamom to your juices.

* *Cayenne Pepper*

Finish off your juice with a dash of cayenne. The heat factor in cayenne pepper is caused by capsaicin, a substance found to help relieve aches and soreness. Adding the spice to your daily diet may help manage appetite and burn more calories after meals, especially if you do not regularly consume it, according to research from Purdue University.

* *Cinnamon*

This popular sweet spice contains iron, calcium, manganese, and even fiber. According to the World's Healthiest Foods website, cinnamon may help lower blood sugar and aid with weight loss by signaling your body not to store sugar, which ultimately may turn to fat. If you have more balanced blood sugar levels, you are also less likely to go through a cycle of sugar highs and lows that make you crave more sugar, and thus lead to more fat. A pinch of ground cinnamon may be added to juices.

* *Coriander*

Coriander is made from dried cilantro seeds and has a spicy, citrus-like flavor. For optimal freshness, use whole coriander seeds and grind them into a powder with a mortar and pestle.

* *Cumin*

A staple in Mediterranean, Asian, African, and Latin American cooking, this pungent spice is known to help improve digestion.

According to the doctors at SportCo Rehabilitation, its distinctive flavor also may increase body temperature, which boosts your metabolism and helps burn calories. Use a touch of ground cumin in juices.

- *Garlic*

Garlic has many health benefits, including antibiotic, immune-enhancing, anticancer, cholesterol-lowering, blood-pressure-reducing, and detoxification-enhancement properties. Fresh garlic is much more potent than cooked or dried and may be easily included in fresh juices.

- *Ginger*

In both its fresh and powder form, ginger is an intense spice well known for its myriad health, anti-inflammatory, and anti-nausea effects. The strength of fresh ginger varies depending on its age and variety. Younger ginger tends to be less spicy than the more readily available mature ginger. Juice fresh ginger first and then add the other ingredients to the machine. This will help squeeze out as much of the ginger juice as possible.

- *Ginseng*

The two most common species of ginseng are Asian and American, and most grocery stores carry American ginseng. Ginseng's active components are called ginsenosides, which are believed to enhance the body's endocrine system and sympathetic nervous system as well as promote relaxation.

- *Nutmeg*

This sweet spice is high in fiber and manganese, which are catalysts for breaking down fats and cholesterol—an important process for weight loss. Purchase ground nutmeg or whole nutmeg and grate as needed.

◆ *Turmeric*

Mildly flavored turmeric is a bright orange root related to ginger. Turmeric has been shown to have anti-inflammatory properties and is believed to be effective against cardiovascular disease, cancer, and diseases that speed aging, such as Alzheimer's and metabolic disorder. When possible, opt for fresh turmeric root, which is now available in many stores, and grate as needed. If you can't find fresh, use turmeric that has been dried and ground.

FREQUENTLY ASKED QUESTIONS

1. *Should I peel fruits and vegetables before juicing them?*

Peel all citrus fruit, including oranges, grapefruit, lemons, and limes, as the skins taste bitter and are high in acid. Leave some of the thick white pith inside the peel on the fruit since it is rich in bioflavonoids and vitamin C. Also, make sure to peel all nonorganic fruit and vegetables, especially carrots and cucumbers.

2. *Can I use a blender instead of a juicer?*

Blenders do not remove the fiber from the juice. One of the points of a juice cleanse is to give your body relief from digesting regular food for a few days. A juicer makes preparing juices much easier, but if you have only a blender, then blend all the ingredients together and strain the juice through a nut milk bag. Discard the pulp.

3. *How do I get enough liquid from the leafy vegetables?*

Some of the leafy vegetables don't have that much juice in them. To get the most juice out of leafy greens, fold them up or wrap them around a cucumber or carrot.

4. *On a juice cleanse, where does my protein come from?*

Vegetables do contain protein, although the amounts are small. For example, 1 cup of spinach has about 1 gram of protein, and 2 cups of broccoli have about 2 grams. Since the length of a juice cleanse is short, missing out on protein will not be a major concern. However, you may add a scoop of vegetable-based, unflavored protein power to your juices to increase the protein content. (See the meal plans in chapter 5 for more information.)

5. *Should I remove seeds and pits? What about stems and leaves?*

Many seeds may be left in the fruit. However, you should always remove hard pit seeds such as those in peaches, plums, and cherries. You don't need to remove stems and leaves, as they are rich in nutrients. The exceptions are carrot tops and rhubarb greens, which should not be juiced.

6. *Can I use prewashed produce?*

Yes, but read the label. Many packaged produce items are prewashed and ready to eat, while some will say that the vegetables must be washed before using.

7. *Should I take supplements during a cleanse?*

Many supplements should be taken with food; taking these supplements with only juice can result in stomach problems. Furthermore, taking supplements while juicing is usually not necessary, because during your juice cleanse you will be drinking so many vitamins, minerals, and nutrients that supplements become redundant. Give your regular supplements a break during your juice cleanse.

8. *How can I "chew my food" if I'm drinking juice?*

Part of chewing your food is to help extract nutrients before swallowing. It also helps you enjoy the flavors and the act of eating. Since you can't chew juice, swish it around in your mouth before swallowing. This slows down the process of drinking your juice, so you can enjoy and savor the experience, and see your juice not just as a drink that you down in a few seconds but as a regular meal.

9. *Can I substitute frozen fruits and vegetables for fresh ones?*

According to a University of Georgia study, some frozen versions of fruit and vegetables are not only cheaper than the fresh versions but may have higher nutritional quality compared to produce that has been stored and shipped before arriving at your table days after it was harvested. The frozen option of many fruits and vegetables can be a budget-friendly, healthy choice when you need to stock up. Check your juicer's user manual or manufacturer's website to see if your machine can handle frozen produce. If not, make sure to thaw it before juicing.

10. *What if I am allergic or do not like a particular fruit or vegetable?*

If you find an ingredient in a recipe that you cannot eat or do not like, replace it with a similar fruit or vegetable. For example, blueberries instead of apples, or beets in place of zucchini. There are so many choices, you can always find a suitable replacement. That is one of the great benefits of a juice cleanse—the almost endless variety of juices you can create.

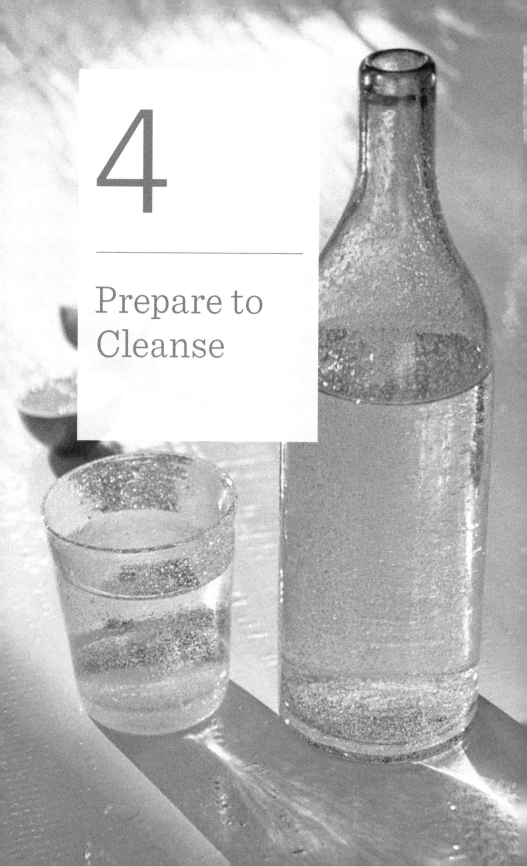

4

Prepare to Cleanse

Let thy food be thy medicine and medicine be thy food.
—Hippocrates

A juice cleanse takes preparation and planning. It is not something you jump into it. There are many decisions to make before undergoing a juice cleanse, such as determining the duration and your ultimate goal as well as preparing your life and environment to support you and your cleanse. If you do not take the time and effort to plan ahead, you won't enjoy the full benefits of your juice cleanse. You may get frustrated with the process, or worse, give up before you finish.

You need to fully understand what you could encounter during your cleanse. While no two people will have the same experience, you should be familiar with the range of emotions and situations you may encounter. This way you will be better prepared to deal with the ups and downs that occur.

WHAT YOU NEED TO KNOW BEFORE YOU CLEANSE

Keep in mind that a juice cleanse is not for everyone. Before you commit, make sure you are aware of the possible reactions you may experience. Potential side effects vary depending on your current and past health conditions, present eating habits, and possible illnesses.

Everyone is different, but many people experience any or some of the following: headaches, achy joints, acne, fatigue, dizziness, sinus problems, low energy, and body odor. The duration and severity of these symptoms may vary, too; they may come and go, or appear once and then vanish. Women may also encounter changes in their menstrual cycles: for example, shorter cycles, or a heavier or lighter flow than usual.

Do not be surprised if your juice cleanse brings back past conditions. This is often a result of toxins being stirred up in the body. For example, some former cigarette smokers have reported tasting cigarettes in their mouth. As mentioned, you may experience withdrawal symptoms from cutting out ingredients like sugar and caffeine, but don't be alarmed. These are signs that your body is cleansing itself, and they will soon pass.

You also might lose some muscle mass by the end of your cleanse. During a cleanse, your body goes into a negative nitrogen balance from the absence of adequate protein. Since you won't be consuming enough protein to maintain your current muscle mass, the body may begin to break down muscle. Do not be too concerned with this. Any muscle lost during a short-term juice cleanse will return once you resume normal eating and exercise.

Finally, for cleanses lasting three to five days, you may find that one day is easier while another is more difficult, with more cravings and headaches. If you're really uncomfortable, drink juices for just one or two meals and eat raw vegetables and fruits for your other meals. If you initially try a longer cleanse (five or seven days) and find it too ambitious, you may shorten it and begin again at a later date. Don't become discouraged; sometimes you need to build up to a longer juice cleanse.

WHAT TO CONSUME AND WHAT TO ELIMINATE

Prepare for your juice cleanse two to three days beforehand to ease your body into the process, which will help reduce hunger cravings. During this period, eat organic fresh fruits and vegetables (many of the same ones you will use for the juice cleanse), fresh salads made with spinach or spring mixes, raw nuts, almond milk, soy milk, and whole grains like quinoa, millet, oats, and brown rice.

Increase your fluid intake. Drink 16 ounces of hot water with lemon and perhaps some grated ginger each morning. Drink a cup of herbal tea at night. During the day, drink at least eight glasses of water.

Stick to your usual schedule of breakfast, lunch, dinner, and snacks, but make sure your meals are light yet filling. Here are some examples:

- *Breakfast*: steel-cut oatmeal, fresh fruit such as berries, poached organic eggs
- *Lunch*: salads with raw vegetables, vegetable soups, raw nuts, fresh fruit
- *Dinner*: whole grains and raw or steamed vegetables, fresh fruit juice (not pasteurized or processed)
- *Snacks*: ten to fifteen raw almonds; a sliced apple or pear with 1 tablespoon almond or peanut butter; or some carrot, celery and/or cucumber sticks with hummus

At the same time, begin eliminating specific foods, some of which may be weight-gain triggers. These include:

- Alcohol
- Caffeine (coffee, soda, black tea, and chocolate)
- Dairy (milk, cheese, yogurt)
- Gluten (bread, baked goods)
- Processed foods (anything that contains preservatives, coloring, flavoring, and additives)
- Refined sugar

- Red meat (which has more calories and saturated fat than chicken or turkey meat)
- White flour products (pasta, crackers, chips)

If you find it difficult to stop eating all of these items at once, limit your consumption of them for two to three days before your juice cleanse. You may experience some general fatigue and discomfort while your body adjusts to these dietary changes.

Also, prior to your cleanse, limit your exercise to light and non-strenuous activities, such as walking, gentle yoga, and stretching. Your energy levels will drop when you're on a juice cleanse, so you want to prepare your body to utilize less energy.

CHOOSING THE RIGHT JUICE CLEANSE

What's your intention for your juice cleanse? Yes, you want to lose weight, and that is a strong motivator, but think beyond this goal. What else do you hope to accomplish? Do you want to change how you eat? Perhaps you want to get healthy, or your goal is to break the habit of eating junk food. You might also want to have more energy or just feel better. When you view your health beyond weight loss, you create a stronger connection to your overall health and wellness and are more likely to reach your goals.

What length juice cleanse should you follow? Optimal cleanse duration is a personal decision; choose the one that best fits your personal schedule and lifestyle. For instance, a one-day cleanse might be ideal if you have trouble setting aside three days for a longer one. A three-day cleanse is best if you have a free three-day weekend, while a five- or seven-day cleanse might be best suited for when you can take time off work and/or your weekly schedule is light and free of obligations and other distractions.

WARNINGS AND PRECAUTIONS

Certain individuals should be careful with a juice cleanse and make sure they first consult with their health care practitioner before attempting one. It never hurts to check in with a professional before beginning any new health practice. Specifically, if you take medication, are pregnant, or have diabetes or kidney disease, check with your doctor before proceeding.

* *Medication.* If you are currently taking any kind of medication, make sure to check with your physician before beginning a juice cleanse. Certain foods may interfere with the efficacy of some medications. For example, WebMD warns that if you are taking statins, antihistamines, blood pressure drugs, psychiatric drugs, pain medications, and immune suppressants, you may have to avoid grapefruit and other citrus fruit juice. According to the Mayo Clinic website, problems may arise because the fruit chemicals may interfere with enzymes in your digestive system that break down the medicine. When that happens, the medication may not stay in your body long enough—or may stay too long.

* *Pregnancy.* On a juice cleanse, you increase your usual amounts of fluids, which means you urinate and have bowel movements more frequently. While this is fine under normal circumstances, a juice cleanse is not recommended if you are pregnant or breastfeeding, as you increase your risk of dehydration. This could affect the fetus as well as your milk production. Also, during pregnancy and lactation, your needs for calcium, protein, and iron are doubled, and you have more need for almost all other nutrients, too. A juice cleanse significantly cuts down on your intake of protein as well as lowers the usual amounts of other nutrients your body demands.

- *Diabetes.* People who have type 1 or type 2 diabetes should not try a juice cleanse. According to the *Huffington Post*, drinking fruit juice means consuming high amounts of fruit sugar, which can cause blood-sugar levels to spike. These spikes are particularly dangerous for people with diabetes and can result in common diabetic symptoms like blurry vision, excessive hunger and thirst, and wounds or infections that heal slowly.

- *Kidney disease.* According to the National Institutes of Health, people with kidney disease have to worry about high levels of potassium in their blood. Many fruits and vegetables used in a juice cleanse contain high amounts of potassium, which can be dangerous for those with kidney disease. Also, people who have begun dialysis need to eat more protein than a juice cleanse allows. Finally, those with advanced kidney disease need to limit their fluid intake, which makes a juice cleanse not recommended.

CLEANSING TIPS TO GET YOU STARTED

Once you've made the decision to do a juice cleanse, it's time to prepare physically and also to get in the right mindset. Here are a few tips to help you sail through a juice cleanse.

- Schedule your cleanse over a weekend or take time off from work and clear your calendar of all commitments, since your energy levels will be lower than usual and you will want to restrict movement as much as possible. You might also experience side effects like headaches and body odor, so ensuring you are in a comfortable environment will help make your juice cleanse a success.

Not-So-Special Occasions

A juice cleanse is an opportunity to make lasting changes; it is not intended to address short-term weight-loss goals for specific events, such as losing ten or twenty pounds for a wedding, vacation, or class reunion. The intention of a juice cleanse is to break bad eating habits, introduce healthier ones, and clean your body of toxins and waste. Do not follow a juice cleanse during an emotionally intense time or major life transition. You do not want emotionally fraught circumstance to drive your cleanse; plus they may distract you during the process. A cleanse should also never be used to bounce back after overindulging. It is not designed to "clean up" a weekend or a vacation of overeating.

- Give your body and brain a break. Since your energy levels will be diminished, you do not want to undertake anything that could cause you to overexert yourself or that normally requires your full attention. This means no work projects, no paying bills, no household chores, and no social engagements. Take care of any errands or shopping beforehand. This way, when your cleanse begins, you can focus on you and your body.

- Keep a journal to record your feelings—physical and emotional—before, during, and after the cleanse. This is a strong support tool to help you manage your thoughts, feelings, and emotions as they emerge.

- Let friends and family know you're planning a juice cleanse and won't be able to go out to dinner or meet up for cocktails. Keeping them informed will help with support and prevent any distractions.

- Meditate or sit quietly for at least ten minutes a day leading up to your cleanse, so it becomes a familiar routine. You may rely on this practice of quiet reflection many times during your cleanse. If this practice is difficult for you, listen to guided meditation recordings.

- Create an environment that is supportive and relaxing. Eliminate any messes or visual reminders of chores, such as piles of dirty dishes and loads of laundry. Your space should be clean, tranquil, and comfortable.

- Collect your favorite gentle music, books you have been meaning to read, and movies you've wanted to watch. Make the experience as much about you as possible. The more support you provide your body, the easier your juice cleanse experience will be.

- Give your skin a daily dry brush to prep it for detoxing. This is a great way to boost blood circulation, which helps remove impurities under the skin. Do this for a few minutes before you shower. Using long sweeps, begin at your toes and work up your legs, then your chest. Then begin from the tips of your fingers and sweep toward your chest again. Finally, sweep your neck and back.

Health and Safety

To ensure that your juices are safe and healthful, follow these steps when making all your juices.

* Wash your hands for at least twenty seconds with soap and warm water before and after preparation.

* Before juicing or eating produce, remove any damaged or bruised areas. Discard any fruit or vegetables that looks past its prime.

* Wash all produce with cool, not warm, water. This includes produce grown organically or purchased from a grocery store or farmers' market.

* Scrub firm produce, especially melons and cucumbers, with a clean brush designated specifically for this purpose.

* Even if the produce requires peeling, such as citrus fruits like oranges, grapefruit, lemons, and limes, wash it first so dirt and bacteria aren't transferred from the knife to the fruit or vegetable.

* Dry produce with a clean cloth towel or paper towel to remove any dirt that may remain after the produce is washed.

* Store fruits and vegetables away from meat, poultry, or seafood, and prevent cross-contamination by not allowing produce to come into contact with kitchen utensils used for those products.

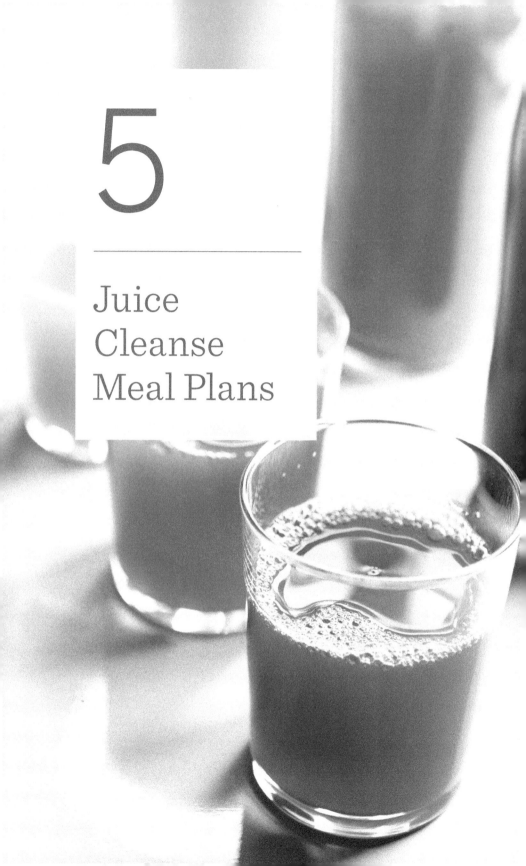

5

Juice Cleanse Meal Plans

The ideal technique for successful fasting is the use of fresh, raw fruit and vegetable juices. On such a diet, the full spectrum of nutrients is supplied in an easily assimilated form, so the digestive tract is able to remain essentially at rest. It is only through the combined use of both cleansing processes and a very good diet that one will be able to reach her or his maximum level of physical health and an unclouded consciousness.
—Rudolph Ballentine, MD, *Diet and Nutrition*

A successful juice cleanse is based on structure and routine. Your daily meal plans will outline exactly what to juice and drink for every meal. This removes any guesswork and eliminates any major decision making so your cleanse will be as stress-free and simple as possible.

A DAY IN THE LIFE OF A JUICE CLEANSER

It is important that you follow some basic juice cleansing guidelines so your cleanse is a success. First, drink six juices a day—one for breakfast, lunch, and dinner, and three for snacks. The juices should be spaced out so you drink one every two hours. Your daily juice schedule will look like this.

- *Breakfast*: within 1 hour of waking
- *Midmorning Snack*: 2 to 3 hours after breakfast
- *Lunch*: 2 to 3 hours after midmorning snack
- *Afternoon Snack*: 2 to 3 hours after lunch
- *Dinner*: 2 to 3 hours after afternoon snack
- *Snack*: at least 2 hours before bedtime

Here are some other guidelines to follow:

* Before drinking your breakfast juice, begin each morning by drinking 8 ounces of warm water with fresh lemon juice and perhaps some freshly grated ginger.

* Drink your last juice snack of the day around 8:00 p.m., or about two hours before bedtime.

* Before bedtime, drink some caffeine-free herbal tea, such as chamomile, rooibos, or mint.

* Do not drink more than six juices per day.

* Fresh is always best when it comes to juicing. Drink your juice immediately; juice begins to lose its nutrients once it is exposed to oxygen, much like sliced apples or avocados quickly turn brown. According to Ann Louise Gittleman, author of *The Fast Track Detox Diet*, vitamins and minerals in a juice can begin to dissipate within fifteen minutes. If you cannot drink the juice within this fifteen-minute period, refrigerate it in an opaque, airtight container for up to twenty-four hours. Don't make it a habit of preparing your juices ahead of time.

* Drink slowly. Swishing the liquid before swallowing helps increase nutrition absorption and satiety. Take your time and enjoy your juice and the moment.

CREATE YOUR OWN JUICE CLEANSING MEAL PLANS

The recipes in this book are set up so you can create your own juice cleanse by following the six-juices-a-day guideline outlined previously. Your selection of juices will be organized this way:

- Breakfast from chapter 7 (Morning Kick-Starters)
- Lunch from chapter 11 (All-Day Essentials)
- Dinner from chapter 13 (Green Energy Boosters)
- Three snacks from chapters 7 through 16

How long your cleanse lasts depends on your personal schedule. Many people enjoy a single-day cleanse as a means to ease into the process and to help better adapt to potential side effects. Others plan a two- or three-day cleanse over a weekend, which is often ideal for people with busy work lives. Many people take on a five- or seven-day cleanse after trying a shorter cleanse. Long-term juice cleanses, such as those longer than 10 days, have the potential to interrupt electrolyte balances and cause major blood sugar spikes that may stress the pancreas. You also run the risk of losing higher amounts of muscle mass since your body will be deprived of adequate protein. Be sure to listen to your body throughout your cleanse and choose what is right for your body as not all cleanses are right for everyone.

No matter which duration you choose, you no doubt will enjoy many of the benefits a juice cleanse offers, especially the desire to change your eating habits, cleanse your body of toxins, and propel your body into the direction of lasting weight loss.

The Cleanses

When setting out to follow a new health regimen, the key to success is deciding on a plan and sticking to it. The following pages detail four specific juice cleanses to help you cleanse and lose weight:

+ 1-Day Revive Cleanse
+ 3-Day Metabolism Boost
+ 5-Day Detox Diet
+ 7-Day Life Transformer

Each plan has a particular objective and is designed to best match specific personal lives and goals. You'll find an explanation of who would most benefit from each plan, each plan's specific goals and tips for success, and finally, a daily meal-by-meal menu and shopping list.

1-Day Revive Cleanse

Cleanser profile: This cleanse is designed for people who want to refresh their digestive system and take a break from their usual diet, but who do not have the time or willpower for a longer cleanse.

Benefits: A one-day cleanse shows how easy it is to eliminate problem foods that contribute to weight gain while giving your digestive system a much-needed break. This plan lets you identify possible side effects and obstacles you may encounter during a longer cleanse.

Warnings: Your body will not experience many of the benefits of a juice cleanse in just one day, and it will not lead to weight loss.

MEAL PLAN

Breakfast: Cucumber, Celery, and Carrot Cleanser
Lunch: Swiss Chard, Apple, and Fennel Swirl
Dinner: Leafy Kale, Bok Choy, and Lime Tonic
Snacks*: Fig, Fennel, and Orange Cocktail ➤

Repeat this snack throughout the day or add one or more from one of the other chapters. The shopping list reflects the meal plan recipes only.

1-Day Revive Cleanse

Coriander, fresh (1 bunch)
Tarragon, fresh (1 bunch)
Apple, Golden Delicious (1)
Figs, fresh (6)
Lime (1)
Oranges, navel (3)
Bok choy, baby (3)
Carrots (2)
Celery (1 bunch)
Cucumbers (4)
Fennel bulbs (6)
Kale, dinosaur (1 bunch)
Swiss chard (1 bunch)

3-Day Metabolism Boost Cleanse

Cleanser profile: Three days is the perfect duration for most people. This cleanse may be done over a long weekend, and you will achieve many of the main benefits of a cleanse. This cleanse is ideal for those looking to break their dependency on unhealthful food and set in motion the ability to lose weight and maintain weight loss.

Benefits: A three-day cleanse enhances your digestive system by flushing out built-up toxins and waste, and increases your metabolism so you begin burning more fat. You will also give your detox system a well-deserved rest and learn how to change your eating habits. You will likely lose a few pounds by the end, with the amount depending on your starting weight, age, and gender.

Warnings: You may experience common cleanse side effects, such as headaches, achy joints, acne, fatigue, dizziness, sinus problems, low energy, and body odor, and your body may not have fully adapted before you finish your cleanse.

MEAL PLAN

Day 1

Breakfast: Red Raspberry, Kale, and Lime Splash
Lunch: Herbed Turnip Greens and Tomato Splash
Dinner: Wheatgrass, Peas, and Mint Cooler
Snacks*: Plum, Arugula, and Strawberry Juice ➤

Repeat this snack throughout the day or add one or more from one of the other chapters. The shopping list reflects the meal plan recipes only.

Day 2

Breakfast: Blueberry-Spinach Cooler
Lunch: Carrot, Lime, and Celery Cocktail
Dinner: Green Apple, Spinach, and Avocado Blend
Snacks*: Sweet Pear and Cauliflower Punch

Day 3

Breakfast: Papaya-Ginger Booster
Lunch: Spinach, Cucumber, and Minty Beet Juice
Dinner: Radicchio, Celery, and Bell Pepper Punch
Snacks*: Cantaloupe and Cranberry Swig

Repeat this snack throughout the day or add one or more from one of the other chapters. The shopping list reflects the meal plan recipes only.

3-Day Metabolism Boost Cleanse

Black peppercorn
Oregano, dried
Cilantro, fresh (1 bunch)
Ginger, fresh
Mint, fresh (1 bunch)
Apple, Granny Smith (1)
Avocado (1)
Blueberries (1 cup)
Cantaloupe (1)
Cranberries (1½ cups)
Lime (1)
Papaya (1)
Pears, red-skinned (3)
Plums, red or purple (12)
Raspberries (2 cups)
Strawberries (3 cups)
Arugula (6 cups)
Beet (1)
Bell pepper, green (1)

Carrots (2)
Cauliflower (3 heads)
Celery (2 bunches)
Cucumbers (2)
Kale, dinosaur (1 bunch)
Lettuce, iceberg (3 heads)
Peas (1 cup)
Radicchio (¾ cup)
Spinach (6 cups)
Tomatoes (2)
Turnip greens (2 cups)
Wheatgrass greens (1 cup)
Coconut water,
    unflavored (½ cup)
Flaxseed, ground (1 tablespoon)
Water, spring (1 cup)
Wheatgrass powder (optional)
    (1 teaspoon)

5-Day Detox Cleanse

Cleanser profile: It is best if you have already tried either the one- or three-day cleanses before attempting the 5-Day Detox Cleanse. On this five-day cleanse, you will begin to lose weight from burning fat, and set in motion a more aggressive and lasting weight-loss strategy.

Benefits: A five-day cleanse allows your body to completely flush toxins, and it will break your dependency on foods that led to your weight gain. Your body's detox system will have the opportunity to rest and renew so it can function at an optimal level and begin eliminating stored fat. You will experience noticeable weight loss—the amount varies depending on your starting weight, age, and other factors. Having given your body a break, when you reintroduce food, you might also be able to identify foods to which you are sensitive or allergic.

Warnings: Since this cleanse is longer than the others, you may have lower levels of energy than on shorter cleanses. You also may encounter more side effects because of its length.

MEAL PLAN

Day 1

Breakfast: Blackberry, Celery, and Banana Blend
Lunch: Rutabaga, Peach, and Swiss Chard Sublime
Dinner: Beet and Basil Cooler
Snacks*: Kiwi, Celery, and Banana Splash

Day 2

Breakfast: Pink Grapefruit, Radish, and Mint Juice
Lunch: Zucchini, Arugula, and Radish Tonic
Dinner: Kohlrabi, Scallion, and Parsley Punch
Snacks*: Blueberry-Cucumber Punch

Day 3

Breakfast: Sunshine Spinach Juice
Lunch: Cinnamon and Sweet Potato Toddy
Dinner: Mustard Greens, Corn, and Celery Splash
Snacks*: Bell Pepper, Carrot, and Tangerine Juice ➤

Repeat this snack throughout the day or add one or more from one of the other chapters. The shopping list reflects the meal plan recipes only.

Day 4

Breakfast: Raspberry and Spinach Morning Toddy
Lunch: Celery, Cantaloupe, and Cauliflower Blend
Dinner: Brussels Sprouts and Cayenne Cocktail
Snacks*: Watermelon and Spinach Cooler

Day 5

Breakfast: Strawberry, Collard Greens, and Ginger Juice
Lunch: Radishes, Corn, and Bell Pepper Blast
Dinner: Collard Greens, Zucchini, and Beet Toddy
Snacks*: Fig, Fennel, and Orange Cocktail

Repeat this snack throughout the day or add one or more from one of the other chapters. The shopping list reflects the meal plan recipes only.

Black peppercorn

Cayenne pepper

Cinnamon, ground

Oregano, dried

Salt

Basil, fresh (1 bunch)

Cilantro, fresh (1 bunch)

Ginger, fresh

Mint, fresh (1 bunch)

Parsley, fresh (1 bunch)

Apples (2)

Bananas, under-ripe (4)

Blackberries (1 cup)

Blueberries (3 cups)

Cantaloupe (1)

Figs, fresh (6)

Grapefruit, pink (1)

Kiwis (6)

Lemon (1)

Oranges, navel (3)

Peach (1)

Raspberries (2 cups)

Strawberries (1 cup)

Tangerines (3)

Watermelon (3 cups)

Arugula (2 cups)

Beet (1)

Bell pepper, green (1)

Bell peppers, red (6)

Brussels sprouts (2 cups)

Carrots (5)

Cauliflower (1 cup)

Celery (7 bunches)

Collard greens (3 cups)

Corn, sweet (3 cups)

Cucumbers (8)

Fennel bulbs (6)

Kohlrabi, light green (2)

Lettuce, iceberg (11 cups)

Mustard greens (2 cups)

Peas (2 cups)

Potato, sweet (1)

Radishes (5)

Rutabaga (1)

Scallions (2)

Spinach (10 cups)

Swiss chard (1 cup)

Zucchini (4)

Coconut water, unflavored
   (2 cups)

Flaxseed, powdered
   (2 teaspoons)

7-Day Life Transformer

Cleanser profile: A seven-day cleanse is not designed for a first-timer. However, if you have tried either the one-day or three-day cleanse and had good results, the seven-day plan may be ideal. It is similar to the 5-Day Detox Cleanse in terms of the basic meal plan, but the extra two days can help you fully establish new eating habits. Sometimes people begin to hit their stride around day five of a juice cleanse. They feel great and begin to notice weight loss. This plan allows you to keep that momentum going a bit longer. Since it is based on the five-day cleanse, follow the 5-Day Detox Cleanse meal plan and then add two additional days.

Benefits: The 7-Day Life Cleanse allows you the extra time you may need to fully break your dependency from your normal diet. The additional two days can help identify problem foods that may be related to your weight gain as well as foods that may trigger digestive or other health issues. During this period you will no doubt feel the effects of weight loss; your clothes may feel looser and you may not feel as bloated as when you began. The amount you lose will vary and depends on your starting weight, age, and gender.

Warnings: This is the longest cleanse, and while you have extra time to reap its benefits, you may experience more side effects, especially low energy levels.

MEAL PLAN

Follow the 5-Day Detox Cleanse, then add these final two days.

Day 6

Breakfast: Cucumber, Celery, and Carrot Cleanser
Lunch: Swiss Chard, Apple, and Fennel Swirl
Dinner: Leafy Kale, Bok Choy, and Lime Tonic
Snacks*: Cantaloupe and Cranberry Swig

Day 7

Breakfast: Papaya-Ginger Booster
Lunch: Spinach, Cucumber, and Minty Beet Juice
Dinner: Radicchio, Celery, and Bell Pepper Punch
Snacks*: Fig, Fennel, and Orange Cocktail ➤

Repeat this snack throughout the day or add one or more from one of the other chapters. The shopping list reflects the meal plan recipes only.

7-Day Life Transformer SHOPPING LIST

Black peppercorn

Cayenne pepper

Cinnamon, ground

Coriander, dried

Oregano, dried

Salt

Tarragon, dried

Basil, fresh (1 bunch)

Cilantro, fresh (1 bunch)

Ginger, fresh

Mint, fresh (1 bunch)

Parsley, fresh (1 bunch)

Apples, Golden Delicious (3)

Bananas, under-ripe (4)

Blackberries (1 cup)

Blueberries (3 cups)

Cantaloupes (2)

Cranberries (1½ cups)

Figs, fresh (12)

Grapefruit, pink (1)

Kiwis (6)

Lemon (1)

Lime (1)

Oranges, navel (6)

Papaya (2 cups)

Peach (1)

Raspberries (2 cups)

Strawberries (1 cup)

Tangerines (3)

Watermelon (3 cups)

Arugula (2 cups)

Beets (2)

Bell peppers, green (2)

Bell peppers, red (6)

Bok choy, baby (3 cups)

Brussels sprouts (2 cups)

Carrots (7)

Cauliflower (1 cup)

Celery (9 bunches)

Collard greens (3 cups)

Corn, sweet (3 cups)

Cucumbers (14)

Fennel bulbs (14)

Kale, dinosaur (1 bunch)

Kohlrabi, light green (2)

Lettuce, iceberg (17 cups)

Mustard greens (2 cups)

Peas (2 cups)

Potato, sweet (1)

Radicchio (¾ cup)

Radishes (5)

Rutabaga (1)

Scallions (2)

Spinach (12 cups)

Swiss chard (3 cups)

Zucchini (4)

Coconut water,
    unflavored (2½ cups)

Flaxseed, powdered
    (2 teaspoons)

Fighting Hunger

You will benefit most from your cleanse by following the meal plans as closely as possible. However, if you are faced with real hunger, eat one of the following:

1 cup warm vegetable broth

A few celery sticks

8 raw almonds

A few cucumber slices

½ cup herbal tea

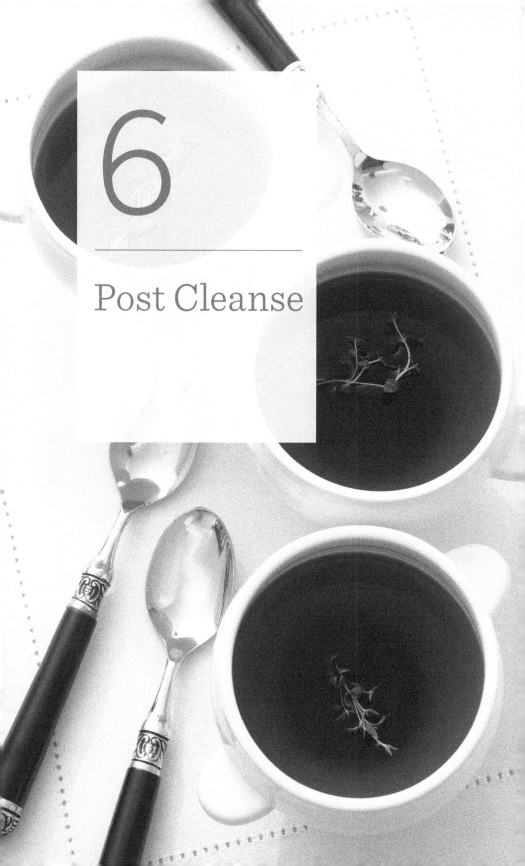

6

Post Cleanse

Fasting is the single greatest natural healing therapy. It is nature's ancient, universal 'remedy' for many problems. ... Juice fasting is commonly used (rather than water alone) as a mild and effective cleansing plan; this is suggested by myself and other doctors and authors, and by many of the European fasting clinics. Fresh juices are easily assimilated and require minimum digestion, while they supply many nutrients and stimulate our body to clear its wastes. Juice fasting is also safer than water fasting, because it supports the body nutritionally while cleansing and probably even produces a better detoxification and quicker recovery.
—Elson M. Haas, MD, *Staying Healthy with Nutrition*

As you move from your juice cleanse to whole foods, take care not to undo the benefits of your cleanse. You have successfully eliminated built-up toxins, and rested and renewed your body's detox system so it can work more efficiently to eliminate the bad stuff and better absorb nutrients that accelerate your weight loss. And best of all, you have revamped your poor eating habits by breaking your bond with processed, high-fat, high-calorie foods and embraced a diet that emphasizes fat-burning fruits and vegetables and portion control. No matter how much weight you have lost during your cleanse, the key to lasting weight loss is to carry forward those new healthful habits.

WHAT TO EXPECT AFTER A CLEANSE

You may experience a range of feelings and emotions after finishing your juice cleanse. You may want to devour anything and everything in sight—or be nonchalant about eating. Some people feel fatigued, others energized. Your mind may be foggy or focused. No matter how you feel afterward, it is important to take care and caution as you make the transition back into your everyday life.

The most crucial step is how you resume eating meals and snacks. You do not want to erase your results by resuming your old ways. It will feel natural to want to reward yourself with pizza, ice cream, or some other favorite comfort food, but it's important to learn to control those impulses. The best way to guard against potential setbacks is to always have a firm meal plan. Know ahead of time what you're going to eat and when you're going to eat it, with specific meal plans in place.

WHAT TO EAT AFTER A CLEANSE

Eat three meals and two snacks, and drink at least one fresh juice every day for the next three or four days. Your meals should include many nutrients that you avoided during your cleanse, especially protein and fiber. As you did with your cleanse, begin your day by drinking a cup of hot water with lemon and some ginger, and end it with a cup of hot herbal tea at night.

What should you eat? The key is to focus on light foods—no high-fat meats, refined sugar, dairy, or processed foods. Since you haven't eaten solid foods for a while, you do not want to stress your body by eating a lot of heavy foods. Keep everything organic to eliminate adding chemicals or toxins into your just-cleansed body.

This is a wonderful opportunity to eliminate foods like sweets, soda, bread (gluten), caffeine, and alcohol that may have contributed to your weight gain. After your cleanse, you may even notice an improvement in your energy level and digestion from cutting out certain foods like dairy or wheat. This may indicate you have a sensitivity or allergy to these foods. Continue your healthful new eating habits by eliminating or at least reducing your intake of the foods to which you're sensitive or allergic.

The following is a guideline of foods to eat for your meals and snacks after your cleanse.

- **_Fresh juices._** Once your cleanse is over, you may still enjoy any of the cleansing juices as a snack or even as a meal replacement.

- **_Homemade vegetable soups._** Homemade vegetable soups provide a lot of vitamins and minerals, which are often depleted during a juice cleanse. Soups may even help you lose weight, according to a study published in the journal _Physiology and Behavior_. The researchers found that people consumed the fewest total daily calories when they ate soup rather than the same ingredients in solid foods. Avoid processed canned soups, which are high in sodium and additives. Homemade versions are not only healthier but also surprisingly easy to make. The healthy Fresh Vegetable Soup recipe on page 82 is a great basic to get started.

- **_Lean meats._** If you plan to reintroduce meat into your diet, do it slowly. Begin with lean choices, such as chicken, turkey, or seafood. Add limited amounts of lean beef as you progress.

- **_Raw fruits and vegetables._** One of the easiest ways to resume eating food is to begin with the same fruits and vegetables you used for juicing. They are high in water content and contain the fiber your digestive system needs to resume its daily detox and elimination processes. For the first day or so, stick with uncooked vegetables, as they provide vital raw juices and pulp to your system. After that you may introduce cooked varieties.

- **_Raw nuts._** Eat raw (not roasted) cashews, almonds, pistachios, and walnuts. When roasted, nuts are usually processed with oils and excess salt, which are unnecessary and diminish the nutrient quality of the nuts. Nuts are high in fiber and ideal for snacks, as they may help you feel fuller. Even though nuts

Fresh Vegetable Soup

1 teaspoon extra-virgin olive oil
1 medium sweet onion, peeled and chopped
1 garlic clove, minced
3 celery stalks, chopped with greens
2 carrots, peeled and chopped
8 cups low sodium vegetable broth
1 can no-salt diced tomatoes
1 large yam, peeled and diced
2 cups green beans, trimmed and cut into 1-inch pieces
1 can white navy beans, drained and rinsed
½ cup shredded spinach or kale
2 tablespoons chopped fresh thyme
Freshly ground black pepper

In a large stock pot, sauté the onion, garlic, celery, and carrots in the oil on medium heat for about 3 to 4 minutes.

Add the broth, diced tomatoes, and yam.

Bring soup to a boil and then turn down the heat and simmer for 60 minutes or until vegetables are tender.

Add green beans, navy beans, spinach, and thyme to the soup and simmer an additional 3 to 4 minutes.

Season to taste.

_____

Serves 6

are high in calories, the *New York Times* reports that research has found that people may snack on modest amounts (no more than a handful) without the risk of weight gain. In fact, nuts may even help you lose weight.

- *Smoothies.* These blended beverages may be a low-fat snack as well as the occasional meal replacement. Several studies have shown that overweight people who follow a meal-replacement plan (which includes both low-calorie smoothies and meals) lose more weight and keep it off compared to those who follow only a low-calorie diet, reports the website Diets.MD. The key is to make low-calorie smoothies without added sugars, processed ingredients, and pasteurized dairy. Make your own healthful smoothies at home by blending together 1 cup of soy milk or almond milk with 1 cup of chopped fruit and 1 cup of greens, such as spinach or a spring mix.

- *Whole, unprocessed grains.* According to the Preventive Medicine Center, unprocessed whole grains are healthier than processed grains, as they retain all their vitamins and minerals. Cooked brown rice, quinoa, millet, spelt, barley, buckwheat, and amaranth are all great choices.

CLEANSING MAINTENANCE

To maintain your momentum, give your post-cleanse diet the same attention as the cleanse itself. Here are some guidelines to follow as you move forward:

- *Keep it simple.* To ease digestion, avoid eating too many different foods in one meal.

- *Chew your food.* You will be tempted to eat quickly since you have not had solid food in several days. Break down solid food as much as possible so your digestive system doesn't have to work extra hard.

- *Avoid overeating.* Focus on decreasing the amount of food you eat. Cut your usual portion size in half or use smaller plates and bowls to give yourself the visual satisfaction that you are not cheating yourself. You will be amazed how much less food you need to feel full.

- *Keep hydrated.* Drink plenty of water and herbal teas through-out the day and with each meal. Not only will staying hydrated support your detox system, it will also curb hunger.

- *Take a probiotic daily.* Good bacteria keeps your digestive tract healthful.

- *Get seven to eight hours of sleep.* Your body and brain need sleep to burn fat and keep energy up.

- *Congratulate yourself!* Remind yourself of what you have accomplished. Write yourself notes of encouragement and leave them where you'll see them at home and work, or send yourself positive-reinforcement e-mails.

TIPS TO AVOID REGAINING WEIGHT

You no doubt have lost weight and feel lighter now that you've fin-ished your cleanse. Most of this weight loss, however, will be water weight, although some may be from burned fat. Water weight loss may fluctuate as you move from a juice-based diet back to whole foods because of your increase in carbohydrates. When your body stores carbs for future energy needs, four water molecules bond with each carbohydrate molecule. Although fruit and vegetable juices do provide some carbohydrates, they don't provide nearly enough to meet your daily energy needs just to keep your body operating.

The result is that your body dips into its stored carbohydrates and converts them to a usable form of energy during a cleanse. The water molecules break off during this process and are excreted in urine and sweat. And since water is heavy, you lose weight.

However, when the body cannot access enough carbs, it will seek out another source of energy. In this case, fat; it is possible your body also tapped into stored fat for energy during a cleanse.

To help you keep losing weight, you need to increase your activity at the same time you introduce whole foods into your diet. During your juice cleanse you refrained from strenuous exercise. Besides conserving energy, you avoided exercise because of the low levels of protein in a juice cleanse, which prevented your body from burning muscle tissue and allowed it to focus on burning fat. Now, it's time to add some regular exercise to your routine. Adding protein back into your diet will help you gain strength and muscle mass, which may keep your metabolism revved up so you burn more fat. It does not matter what kind of exercise you adopt: weights, yoga, or aerobics. The key is to get moving and stay moving.

Another way to prevent gaining back weight is to do another juice cleanse. Your body will often tell you when it is time, but some signs include poor elimination, fatigue, trouble sleeping, skin problems, and especially cravings for sugar or rich comfort foods. As you continue toward your weight-loss goal or if you're struggling to maintain a goal weight, a juice cleanse may be a tool to get yourself back on track, especially if you fell back into your previous bad habits and began to gain weight. If you reach a plateau on a weight-loss program, a juice cleanse may help you push past it.

To make lasting weight-loss changes, you have to make significant changes that become part of your lifestyle. The first step to weight loss begins when you change your behavior and begin to heal your body. A juice cleanse may get you moving in the right direction.

Part Two

JUICE CLEANSE RECIPES

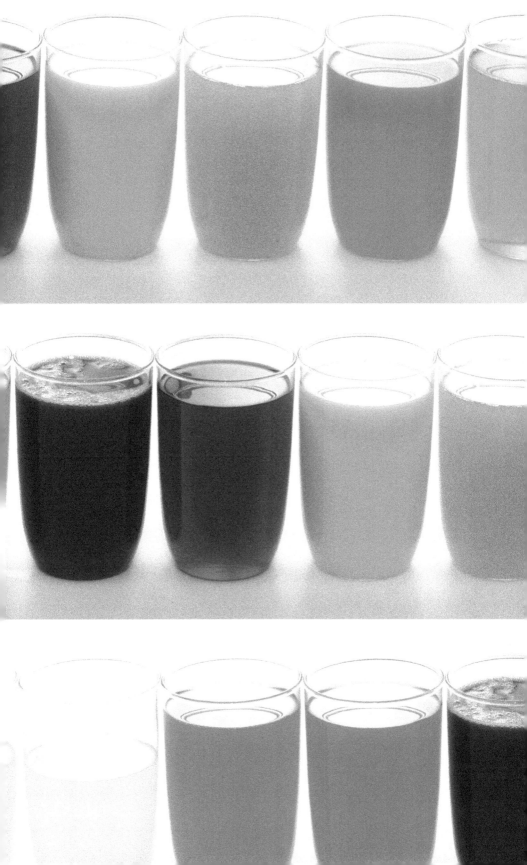

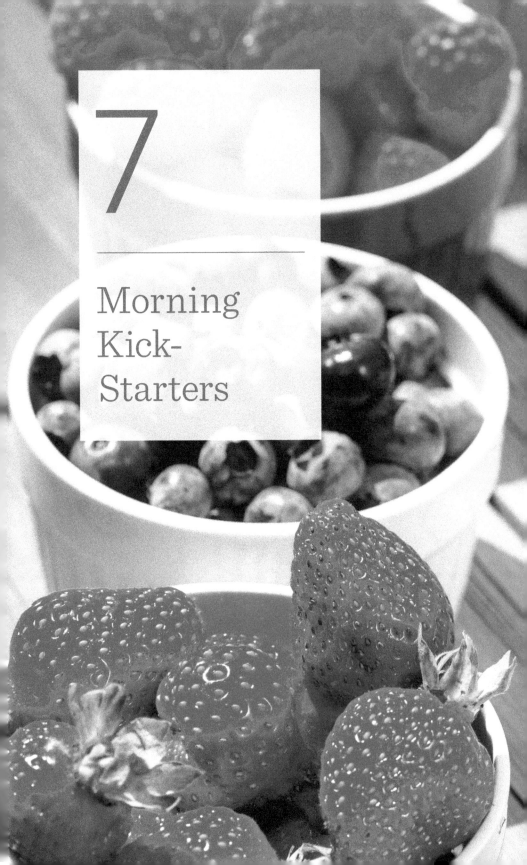

7

Morning Kick-Starters

RECIPES

Cucumber, Celery, and Carrot Cleanser

BONE & BLOOD HEALTH ◆ CLEANSE & DETOX ◆ HEART HEALTH

Per Serving
Calories: 84
Fat: 1 g
Carbs: 24 g
Protein: 4 g
Sugar: 12 g

High in vitamin K, cucumbers also have a high water content and a mild, fresh melon flavor. Celery is rich in vitamin A, and carrots are packed with phytonutrients. This juice is a refreshing way to start to your day. If you find this juice needs a little sweetening, feed one-fourth of an apple through the juicer after the carrots.

2 cucumbers, halved lengthwise
2 celery stalks with leaves
2 carrots

Feed the cucumbers, celery, and carrots through the juicer.

Stir and pour the juice into a glass. Drink immediately.

Serves 1

Celery is a great source of antioxidant nutrients, including vitamin C, beta-carotene, and manganese. It is also an excellent source of vitamin K and good source of folate, potassium, calcium, and vitamins A (in the form of carotenoids), B_2, and B_6. Celery also contains approximately 35 mg of sodium per stalk, so keep this in mind if you are watching your sodium intake or are salt sensitive.

Red Raspberry, Kale, and Lime Splash

ANTI-CANCER ◆ BRAIN HEALTH ◆ HEART HEALTH

Per Serving
Calories: 179
Fat: 4 g
Carbs: 46 g
Protein: 13 g
Sugar: 9 g

Raspberries are high in vitamin C and copper, the latter of which is necessary for collagen production to support tissue repair. They also contain rheosmin, known to increase the metabolism in fat cells. Kale is rich in vitamins A, C, and K. The combined flavors of this juice make it a delicious morning drink.

¼ lime, peeled and seeded
2 cups raspberries
1 cup packed dinosaur kale (leaves and stems)
4 celery stalks with leaves

Feed the lime and raspberries through the juicer, followed by the kale and celery.

Stir and pour the juice into a glass. Drink immediately.

Serves 1

Kale is a true super food. It has one of the highest levels of the powerful antioxidant vitamin K (a whopping 684 percent of the recommended daily value). According to a study in the *American Journal of Clinical Nutrition*, a diet rich in vitamin K may reduce your risk for cancer. Anyone taking anticoagulants, such as warfarin, should check with their doctor or pharmacist about eating kale and other dark, leafy green vegetables.

Tangerine, Fennel, and Parsley Cocktail

ANTI-CANCER ◆ BONE & BLOOD HEALTH ◆ DIGESTIVE HEALTH

Per Serving
Calories: 93
Fat: 1 g
Carbs: 32 g
Protein: 5 g
Sugar: 6 g

Fennel contains the phytonutrient compound anethole, a powerful antioxidant, as well as vitamin C, calcium, potassium, and folate, a B vitamin that protects blood vessel walls from free radicals and helps with blood flow. Parsley is loaded with vitamin K and contains oils shown to inhibit tumor growth. The splash of tangerine makes this juice a refreshing start to the day.

1 tangerine, peeled, seeded, and sectioned
4 fresh parsley sprigs
2 fennel bulbs
2 celery stalks with leaves

Feed the tangerine and parsley through the juicer, followed by the fennel bulbs and celery.

Stir and pour the juice into a glass. Drink immediately.

Serves 1

Tangerines are in season from October to January. There are three types: clementines, tangelos, and temples. Clementines are known for their sweet-tasting juice. Tangelos look like an orange but are smaller and bell shaped. Temple oranges are a hybrid of an orange and a tangerine.

Blueberry-Spinach Cooler

ANTI-CANCER ◆ BRAIN HEALTH ◆ HEART HEALTH

Per Serving
Calories: 67
Fat: 1 g
Carbs: 20 g
Protein: 3 g
Sugar: 13 g

Spinach is one of the world's most nutritious foods. Loaded with vitamins A and K, it's also high in folate, manganese, copper, and magnesium. Antioxidant-rich blueberries are sweet in flavor, helping make this juice sweet. Iceberg lettuce increases the hydration factor because it is packed with water.

2 cups packed spinach
2 cups shredded and packed iceberg lettuce
1 cup blueberries
1 celery stalk with leaves

Feed the spinach and lettuce through the juicer, followed by the blueberries and celery.

Stir and pour the juice into a glass. Drink immediately.

Serves 1

If you don't have time to shred your iceberg lettuce, you can feed half a small head of lettuce through your juicer a couple leaves at a time—it will add up to the same amount. Iceberg lettuce is often overlooked when considering nutritional food, but it is actually packed with important vitamins and minerals. There is 20 percent of the recommended daily allowance (RDA) of vitamin K in 1 cup of iceberg lettuce and 15 percent of the RDA of vitamin A.

Strawberry, Collard Greens, and Ginger Juice

BONE & BLOOD HEALTH ✦ BRAIN HEALTH ✦ HEART HEALTH

Per Serving
Calories: 136
Fat: 6 g
Carbs: 21 g
Protein: 6 g
Sugar: 7 g

Strawberries provide a big boost of vitamin C as do collard greens. Collard greens are also loaded with vitamin K. Ginger is known for its ability to ease indigestion, but it also has powerful antioxidants and anti-inflammatory properties. The flaxseed adds a little protein and fiber.

1 tablespoon peeled and sliced fresh ginger
2 cups packed collard greens
1 cup strawberries
2 cups shredded and packed iceberg lettuce
2 teaspoons powdered flaxseed

Feed all ingredients except the flaxseed through the juicer.

Stir and pour the juice into a glass.

Stir in the flaxseed. Drink immediately.

Serves 1

Pink Grapefruit, Radish, and Mint Juice

ANTI-CANCER ◆ BONE & BLOOD HEALTH ◆ DIGESTIVE HEALTH

Per Serving
Calories: 31
Fat: 0 g
Carbs: 9 g
Protein: 1 g
Sugar: 7 g

Grapefruit's plentiful vitamin C supports the immune system, and the antioxidant lycopene is found in the pink and red varieties. The combination of peppery radishes and cool mint temper the tartness of the grapefruit juice. If you are taking any medication, check with your doctor regarding potential adverse interactions with grapefruit juice.

½ pink grapefruit, peeled, sectioned, and seeded
1 radish
2 tablespoons fresh mint leaves
4 celery stalks with leaves

Feed the grapefruit and radish through the juicer, followed by the mint and celery.

Stir and pour the juice into a glass. Drink immediately.

Serves 1

Raspberry and Spinach Morning Toddy

ANTI-CANCER ◆ BONE & BLOOD HEALTH ◆ HEART HEALTH

Per Serving
Calories: 68
Fat: 2 g
Carbs: 26 g
Protein: 4 g
Sugar: 10 g

Spinach is a nutrient superstar, but it is the bright, tart raspberry flavor that dominates this juice. Packed with vitamins A, C, and K, this is an extra-hydrating breakfast juice. Adding a little of the raspberry pulp to the juice provides even more flavor and some fiber.

2 cups raspberries
2 cups shredded and packed iceberg lettuce
2 cups packed spinach
2 celery stalks with leaves

Feed the raspberries through the juicer. Scoop 1 tablespoon of the pulp from the pulp basket and set aside.

Feed the lettuce, spinach, and celery through the juicer.

Stir and pour the juice into a glass.

Add the reserved raspberry pulp to the juice and stir thoroughly. Drink immediately.

Serves 1

Papaya-Ginger Booster

ANTI-CANCER ◆ CLEANSE & DETOX ◆ DIGESTIVE HEALTH

Per Serving
Calories: 144
Fat: 1 g
Carbs: 41 g
Protein: 2 g
Sugar: 28 g

Bursting with vitamins A and C, papaya may help reduce inflammation, says Eric Braverman, author of Younger (Thinner) You Diet. *Coconut water provides extra liquid and potassium. Together, these ingredients make a great taste-of-the-tropics breakfast drink.*

1 tablespoon peeled and sliced fresh ginger
2 cups chopped papaya, peeled and seeded
½ cup unflavored coconut water

Feed the ginger and papaya through the juicer.

Add the coconut water to the juice.

Stir and pour the juice into a glass. Drink immediately.

Serves 1

Ginger has been consumed for centuries for health ailments and is an important ingredient when juicing. It is one of the components used in Joe Cross's morning wake-up drink in the film *Fat, Sick & Nearly Dead* (see the Resources section). Ginger can support weight-loss goals because it improves digestion by stimulating digestive enzymes and increasing the pH in the stomach. Ginger also helps burn fat because it contains a thermogenic agent.

Blackberry, Celery, and Banana Blend

ANTI-CANCER ◆ DIGESTIVE HEALTH ◆ HEART HEALTH

Per Serving
Calories: 107
Fat: 1 g
Carbs: 33 g
Protein: 3 g
Sugar: 1g

Packed with vitamins C and K and the mineral manganese, blackberries make a dramatic-looking juice on their own, but the touch of banana flavor creates a familiar and satisfying breakfast drink. This is not a sweet juice, because you are using an under-ripe banana, so if you like more natural sugar in your morning juice, try adding half an apple instead.

1 cup blackberries
4 celery stalks with leaves
1 slightly under-ripe banana, peeled
½ cup unflavored coconut water

Feed blackberries and celery through the juicer.

Use a blender to combine the banana and coconut water.

Stir and pour the juice into a glass.

Stir the banana mixture into the juice.
Drink immediately.

Serves 1

Carrot-Orange Juice

ANTI-CANCER ◆ DIGESTIVE HEALTH ◆ HEART HEALTH

Per Serving
Calories: 67
Fat: 0 g
Carbs: 21 g
Protein: 1 g
Sugar: 14 g

If you are used to starting your mornings with a glass of orange juice, this recipe won't be too much of a stretch. The carrots enhance the sunny color and add beta-carotene to an already healthful juice. Carrots also can help regulate blood sugar even though they have a glycemic index of 80.

4 carrots
1 orange, peeled and sectioned
1 apple, cored

Feed the carrots, orange, and apple through the juicer.

Stir and pour the juice into 2 glasses. Drink immediately.

Serves 2

Carrots might become your ingredient of choice for many juicing recipes because they add a satisfying sweetness, blend well with other ingredients, and are inexpensive. If budget is not a huge concern, try juicing all the different color carrots available to see the range of gorgeous colors produced. The flavor won't change regardless of the carrot's color.

Tomato-Veggie Juice

ANTI-CANCER ✦ CLEANSE & DETOX ✦ HEART HEALTH

Per Serving
Calories: 34
Fat: 1 g
Carbs: 10 g
Protein: 2 g
Sugar: 6 g

What better way to start your day than with a glass full of healthful nutrients? This juice is packed with antioxidants, vitamins, and minerals from A to Z. It tastes like a salad in a glass.

2 tomatoes, stemmed and halved
2 celery stalks with leaves
1 cup shredded and packed romaine lettuce
1 red bell pepper, cored and seeded
1 carrot
½ cup fresh parsley

Feed the tomatoes through the juicer, followed by the celery and lettuce.

Feed the bell pepper through the juicer, followed by the carrot and parsley.

Stir and pour the juice into 2 glasses. Drink immediately.

Serves 2

Lemon, Parsley, and Pear Juice

ANTI-CANCER ◆ BRAIN HEALTH ◆ HEART HEALTH

Per Serving
Calories: 94
Fat: 1 g
Carbs: 30 g
Protein: 3 g
Sugar: 17 g

This refreshing morning juice has a bit of lemon zing to wake you up and an energy boost from fresh parsley to keep you going. This juice can also be jazzed up with an inch of peeled fresh ginger or a sprig of fresh basil for an interesting flavor change.

4 celery stalks with leaves
2 cups packed baby spinach
2 pears, cored
1 cup fresh parsley
½ lemon, peeled and seeded

Feed the celery through the juicer, followed by the spinach and pears.

Feed the parsley and lemon through the juicer.

Stir and pour the juice into 2 glasses. Drink immediately.

Serves 2

Sunshine Spinach Juice

ANTI-CANCER ◆ DIGESTIVE HEALTH ◆ HEART HEALTH

Per Serving
Calories: 81
Fat: 1 g
Carbs: 25 g
Protein: 2 g
Sugar: 16 g

This juice recipe is aptly named because it will leave you feeling sunny and bright, ready to face the day ahead. Pears provide a quick source of energy because they are high in natural sugars. Both pears and apples are a member of the rose family, so expect a heady sweet fragrance when you cut them.

2 cups packed spinach
2 celery stalks with leaves
2 carrots
2 apples, cored
1 (1-inch) piece fresh ginger, peeled
1/2 lemon, peeled and seeded

Feed the spinach and celery through the juicer.

Feed the carrots, apples, and ginger through the juicer, followed by the lemon.

Stir and pour the juice into 2 glasses. Drink immediately.

Serves 2

Apple, Beet, and Mint Juice

DIGESTIVE HEALTH ◆ CLEANSE & DETOX ◆ HEART HEALTH

Per Serving
Calories: 110
Fat: 1 g
Carbs: 34 g
Protein: 3 g
Sugar: 22 g

One of the benefits of drinking juice for breakfast is that it is easier on your digestive system than whole foods—your body absorbs the nutrients more quickly so you feel the benefits all morning long. The fresh mint in this juice will be a real eye opener and help start your day with a calm digestive system.

5 carrots
2 apples, cored
1 beet, chopped
½ cup fresh mint leaves

Feed the carrots, apples, beet, and mint through the juicer.

Stir and pour the juice into 2 glasses. Drink immediately.

Serves 2

The best mint for this recipe is fresh, preferably from your own garden. When purchasing your mint, make sure there are no brown spots on the leaves and the mint is not wilted. The juice you drink should come from the highest-quality ingredients to ensure the best nutritional value.

Blueberry-Cabbage Juice

DIGESTIVE HEALTH ◆ BRAIN HEALTH ◆ HEART HEALTH

Per Serving
Calories: 72
Fat: 0 g
Carbs: 22 g
Protein: 2 g
Sugar: 14 g

If you like to start your morning with something sweet, skip the toaster pastries and go for this juice. Not only is it packed with vitamins and minerals, but it is sweet and colorful to boot. Strawberries will also work very well with the other ingredients and create a very red juice.

1 cup blueberries
1 cucumber, halved lengthwise
1 apple, cored
1 cup shredded and packed red cabbage

Feed the blueberries through the juicer, followed by the cucumber.

Feed the apple and cabbage through the juicer.

Stir and pour the juice into 2 glasses. Drink immediately.

Serves 2

Blueberries are a super food that is packed full of antioxidants and vitamins B_2, C, and E. They can reduce the risk of developing cancer, Alzheimer's disease, and bladder infections. Try all the different types of blueberries, including wild blueberries if they are available in your area.

Green Apple-Spinach Juice

ANTI-CANCER ◆ DIGESTIVE HEALTH ◆ HEART HEALTH

Per Serving
Calories: 72
Fat: 0 g
Carbs: 22 g
Protein: 1 g
Sugar: 14 g

While you may not be used to your morning glass of apple juice being green, this recipe is better than it looks. Made with power-packed ingredients like spinach and celery, it will have you going all morning long.

1 (1-inch) piece fresh ginger, peeled
2 cups packed baby spinach
2 green apples, cored
2 celery stalks with leaves
1 carrot

Feed the ginger and spinach through the juicer, followed by the apples.

Feed the celery and carrot through the juicer.

Stir and pour the juice into 2 glasses. Drink immediately.

Serves 2

If you want a slightly different version of this juice, substitute parsnip for the carrot. You don't need to peel them, and if the parsnips are too large for your juicer's feed chute, simply chop them into large chunks. Parsnip combines beautifully with the heat of the ginger.

Strawberry-Cucumber Cocktail

ANTI-CANCER ◆ BRAIN HEALTH ◆ HEART HEALTH

Per Serving
Calories: 70
Fat: 0 g
Carbs: 22 g
Protein: 2 g
Sugar: 13 g

If you prefer to start off with something light in the morning, this Strawberry-Cucumber Cocktail is the perfect blend of sweet and refreshing. Depending on the size of the berry, you can just pop them whole in the juicer. Try to get strawberries in season in early summer to experience the sweetest taste.

2 carrots
1 cup halved strawberries
1 cucumber, halved lengthwise
1 pear, cored

Feed the carrots and strawberries through the juicer, followed by the cucumber and pear.

Stir and pour the juice into 2 glasses. Drink immediately.

Serves 2

Pink Grapefruit Juice

ANTI-CANCER ✦ BONE & BLOOD HEALTH ✦ DIGESTIVE HEALTH

Per Serving
Calories: 70
Fat: 0 g
Carbs: 23 g
Protein: 2 g
Sugar: 18 g

Not only is grapefruit juice a surefire way to wake up in the morning, but it also has antiaging benefits. Enjoy this juice to keep your skin healthy and smooth. You can actually feed peeled grapefruit through your juicer if it is sectioned, including the seeds, which contain many nutrients.

2 pink grapefruit, peeled, sectioned, and seeded
4 celery stalks with leaves
1 navel orange, peeled and sectioned

Feed the grapefruit, celery, and orange through the juicer.

Stir and pour the juice into 2 glasses. Drink immediately.

Serves 2

Grapefruit has many health benefits, but it also can also interact quite strongly with many medications; if you are taking medicine, check with your doctor before consuming grapefruit juice. If you are not allowed to have grapefruit, substitute two more oranges and a lemon in this juice. The lemon adds a nice tartness, which mimics the missing grapefruit.

8

Cleansing
Juices

RECIPES

Cucumber-Fennel Detox Juice

ANTI-CANCER ◆ CLEANSE & DETOX ◆ HEART HEALTH

Per Serving
Calories: 74
Fat: 1 g
Carbs: 23 g
Protein: 4 g
Sugar: 9 g

This recipe is full of cleansing ingredients such as cucumber, fennel, celery, and parsley, which can all be very effective when trying to reach weight-loss goals. You won't be disappointed with the taste, either. The fennel adds a lovely licorice taste, and it can be completely juiced, including the feathery fronds on top.

2 celery stalks with leaves
1 cucumber, halved lengthwise
1 fennel bulb, chopped
1 apple, cored
1 cup fresh parsley
½ lemon, peeled and seeded

Feed the celery, cucumber, fennel bulb, and apple through the juicer.

Feed the parsley and lemon through the juicer.

Stir and pour the juice into 2 glasses. Drink immediately.

Serves 2

Broccoli-Beet Juice

ANTI-CANCER ✦ CLEANSE & DETOX ✦ HEART HEALTH

Per Serving
Calories: 94
Fat: 1 g
Carbs: 28 g
Protein: 6 g
Sugar: 15 g

Beets are rich in phytonutrients called betalains, which not only provide antioxidant and anti-inflammatory benefits but also help detoxify the body. These phytonutrients are particularly beneficial for liver detoxification. You can also add the beet greens to this juice after you rinse them well in cool water.

2 beets, chopped
2 broccoli stalks
2 celery stalks with leaves
1 carrot
1 orange, peeled and sectioned
1/2 lemon, peeled and seeded

Feed the beets through the juicer, followed by the broccoli and celery.

Feed the carrot, orange, and lemon through the juicer.

Stir and pour the juice into 2 glasses. Drink immediately.

Serves 2

Blueberry-Kale Juice

BRAIN HEALTH ◆ CLEANSE & DETOX ◆ HEART HEALTH

Per Serving
Calories: 88
Fat: 1 g
Carbs: 19 g
Protein: 5 g
Sugar: 6 g

Blueberries are full of healthful vitamins and minerals, which make them an essential element in a detox. They also give this recipe a sweet, fresh flavor. Kale is also a nutritional powerhouse, so when combined with the blueberries, this juice becomes a must-have addition when you need a boost or you are feeling a bit under the weather.

1 cup blueberries
2 cups packed dinosaur kale (leaves and stems)
2 romaine lettuce leaves
1 celery stalk with leaves

Feed the blueberries through the juicer, followed by the kale.

Feed the lettuce and celery through the juicer.

Stir and pour the juice into 2 glasses. Drink immediately.

Serves 2

Celery-Wheatgrass Juice

BONE & BLOOD HEALTH ✦ BRAIN HEALTH ✦ CLEANSE & DETOX

Per Serving
Calories: 79
Fat: 0 g
Carbs: 21 g
Protein: 3 g
Sugar: 17 g

The key to juicing wheatgrass is to bundle it into a ball and push it through the juicer with a celery stalk. If you don't have a wheatgrass juicer, this will only work with a masticating juicer, so make sure you have the right model before you attempt this recipe.

3 ounces fresh wheatgrass
4 celery stalks with leaves
2 apples, cored
1 cup packed spinach

Ball the wheatgrass into 1 or 2 balls. Feed the balls of wheatgrass through the juicer, using a stalk of celery to push them through.

Feed the remaining celery stalks through the juicer, followed by the apples and spinach.

Stir and pour the juice into 2 glasses. Drink immediately.

Serves 2

Wheatgrass is a nutritional powerhouse and can be consumed by people who are gluten sensitive even though it is a form of wheat. Wheatgrass is one of the best food sources for living chlorophyll, which can help build the blood, fight free radicals, and slow the aging process.

Sweet Romaine-Apple Juice

CLEANSE & DETOX ◆ DIGESTIVE HEALTH ◆ HEART HEALTH

Per Serving
Calories: 116
Fat: 0 g
Carbs: 37 g
Protein: 1 g
Sugar: 27 g

Many people have a hard time sticking to their cleanse because they get bored with the recipes or they find them unpleasant. While this recipe is made with romaine lettuce, all you will taste is the sweetness of apples. The recipe is also very simple, so it makes a great choice for beginner juicer enthusiasts getting familiar with the juicing process.

4 cups shredded and packed romaine lettuce
4 apples, cored

Feed the lettuce through the juicer, followed by the apples.

Stir and pour the juice into 2 glasses. Drink immediately.

Serves 2

Romaine lettuce is a common ingredient in many kitchens, but you might not realize it is also very nutritious. It is an excellent source of vitamins A, C, B_1, and B_2. Make sure you wash every leaf individually, because grit and dirt can hide in the bottoms of the leaves.

Cilantro, Carrot, and Celery Juice

BRAIN HEALTH ◆ CLEANSE & DETOX ◆ HEART HEALTH

Per Serving
Calories: 32
Fat: 1 g
Carbs: 10 g
Protein: 2 g
Sugar: 5 g

Cilantro is a refreshing, flavorful herb that works particularly well in juices. It is also known for its detoxification properties. Cilantro can be a bit of an acquired taste if you are not familiar with its pungent flavor, so try a smaller amount in the recipe until you know you like it.

2 celery stalks with leaves
2 carrots
1 cup fresh cilantro

Feed the celery through the juicer, followed by the carrots and cilantro.

Stir and pour the juice into a glass. Drink immediately.

Serves 1

Basil-Lime Juice

ANTI-CANCER ◆ CLEANSE & DETOX ◆ HEART HEALTH

Per Serving
Calories: 23
Fat: 0 g
Carbs: 7 g
Protein: 1 g
Sugar: 2 g

Not only does lime provide this recipe with its light, refreshing flavor, it also provides powerful detoxification benefits. Limes are a very common ingredient in any store, but for an intense juice experience, try using key limes if you can find them. Key limes are small, thin-skinned immature limes that have an incredibly acidic taste.

1 cucumber, halved lengthwise
2 celery stalks with leaves
2 cups fresh basil
1 lime, peeled, halved, and seeded

Feed the cucumber through the juicer, followed by the celery.

Feed the basil and lime halves through the juicer.

Stir and pour the juice into 2 glasses. Drink immediately.

Serves 2

Apple-Arugula Juice

ANTI-CANCER ◆ BONE & BLOOD HEALTH ◆ CLEANSE & DETOX

Per Serving
Calories: 125
Fat: 1 g
Carbs: 39 g
Protein: 1 g
Sugar: 28 g

Arugula is a bitter green that helps detoxify the body. When arugula is combined with apples, as in this recipe, the apple taste dominates. It is best to use sweeter apples in this juice to offset the flavor of the arugula. Try Red Delicious, Gala, and Honeycrisp varieties rather than McIntoshs or Courtlands.

2 apples, cored
$\frac{1}{2}$ cup packed arugula
1 celery stalk with leaves
$\frac{1}{2}$ lemon, peeled and seeded

Feed the apples through the juicer, followed by the arugula.

Feed the celery stalk and lemon through the juicer.

Stir and pour the juice into a glass. Drink immediately.

Serves 1

Arugula, also known as rocket, is a pretty green color that has powerful disease-fighting nutrients. It is a great source of vitamin K and folic acid. Arugula can promote a healthy immune system and help prevent cancer and Alzheimer's disease.

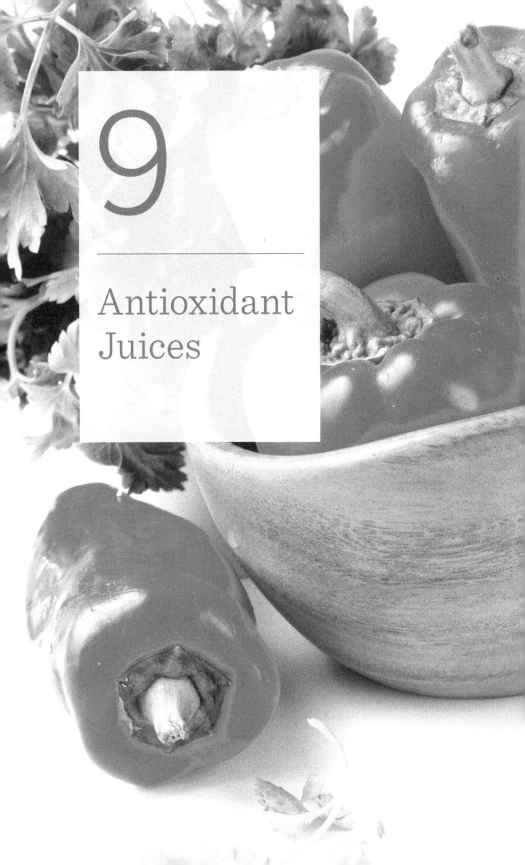

9

Antioxidant Juices

RECITES

Blueberry-Broccoli Juice

ANTI-CANCER ◆ BONE & BLOOD HEALTH ◆ HEART HEALTH

Per Serving
Calories: 81
Fat: 1 g
Carbs: 24 g
Protein: 7 g
Sugar: 9 g

Blueberries are one of the best sources of antioxidants. A single cup of blueberries contains an antioxidant capacity of more than thirteen thousand. This is one of the reasons they are considered to be a super food.

2 celery stalks with leaves
1 head broccoli
1 cup blueberries
½ lemon, peeled and seeded

Feed the celery through the juicer, followed by the broccoli.

Feed the blueberries and lemon through the juicer.

Stir and pour the juice into 2 glasses. Drink immediately.

Serves 2

Cranberry-Artichoke Juice

ANTI-CANCER ◆ CLEANSE & DETOX ◆ DIGESTIVE HEALTH

Per Serving
Calories: 40
Fat: 0 g
Carbs: 14 g
Protein: 3 g
Sugar: 4 g

Cranberries and artichokes may not sound like good juice mates, but you will definitely be a believer after trying this delicious juice. Artichokes are actually a member of the sunflower family and a thistle. Their taste can be bitter, so don't expect this to be a sweet juice.

1 artichoke
1 cucumber, halved lengthwise
1 cup cranberries
1 celery stalk with leaves

Cut off and discard the stem of the artichoke just at the base of the bud. Remove and discard any tough or dry outer leaves.

Pull off the softer inner green leaves of the artichoke and feed them through the juicer in small batches.

Chop the artichoke heart and feed it through the juicer.

Feed the cucumber, cranberries, and celery through the juicer.

Stir and pour the juice into 2 glasses. Drink immediately.

Serves 2

Green Apple-Cucumber Juice

ANTI-CANCER ◆ CLEANSE & DETOX ◆ DIGESTIVE HEALTH

Per Serving
Calories: 71
Fat: 0 g
Carbs: 22 g
Protein: 1 g
Sugar: 15 g

Green apples like Granny Smith contain high levels of antioxidants—more than five thousand per apple. Granny Smith apples also brown slower than other apples due to a higher acid content. This means your juice will have a refreshing tartness.

2 romaine lettuce leaves
2 green apples, cored
1 celery stalk with leaves
1 cucumber, halved lengthwise

Feed the lettuce through the juicer, followed by the apples, celery, and cucumber.

Stir and pour the juice into 2 glasses. Drink immediately.

Serves 2

Tomato Gazpacho Juice

BRAIN HEALTH ◆ CLEANSE & DETOX ◆ HEART HEALTH

Per Serving
Calories: 37
Fat: 1 g
Carbs: 11 g
Protein: 3 g
Sugar: 5 g

When you think of antioxidants, you probably think of fruit. Tomatoes are also a fruit and are rich in a certain antioxidant called lycopene. Lycopene is actually more abundant when tomatoes are cooked but still provide plenty of disease-fighting punch in this recipe. Garlic is also incredibly high in antioxidants, so try this juice when you are fighting a cold or feeling run-down.

4 plum tomatoes, halved
1 green bell pepper, cored and seeded
1 cucumber, halved lengthwise
1 cup fresh cilantro
1 garlic clove

Feed the tomatoes through the juicer, followed by the bell pepper and cucumber.

Feed the cilantro and garlic through the juicer.

Stir and pour the juice into 2 glasses. Drink immediately.

Serves 2

Apple, Pecan, and Cinnamon Juice

ANTI-CANCER ◆ CLEANSE & DETOX ◆ HEART HEALTH

Per Serving
Calories: 263
Fat: 21 g
Carbs: 25 g
Protein: 5 g
Sugar: 16 g

In addition to being full of flavor, pecans are also a great source of antioxidants. In this recipe, they are flavored with a hint of cinnamon. This juice is like apple crumble in a glass.

2 green apples, cored
1 cucumber, halved lengthwise
1 celery stalk with leaves
1 romaine lettuce leaf
¼ cup raw pecans
¼ teaspoon ground cinnamon

Feed the apples, cucumber, celery, and lettuce through the juicer.

In a blender, combine the juice, pecans, and cinnamon. Blend on high speed for 30 to 60 seconds, or until smooth.

Pour the juice into 2 glasses. Drink immediately.

Serves 2

Strawberry-Kale Juice

ANTI-CANCER ◆ BRAIN HEALTH ◆ HEART HEALTH

Per Serving
Calories: 60
Fat: 1 g
Carbs: 15 g
Protein: 4 g
Sugar: 4 g

Kale is a good source of both vitamins A and C, and it also contains the antioxidant lutein, which is essential for eye health. Carrots are also very good for vision due to their beta-carotene content. So this juice packs a double nutrient whammy.

6 kale leaves
2 celery stalks with leaves
1 carrot
1 cup halved strawberries
½ lemon, peeled and seeded

Feed the kale through the juicer, followed by the celery.

Feed the carrot through the juicer, followed by the strawberries and lemon.

Stir and pour the juice into 2 glasses. Drink immediately.

Serves 2

Radical Red Bell Pepper Juice

ANTI-CANCER • DIGESTIVE HEALTH • HEART HEALTH

Per Serving
Calories: 60
Fat: 0 g
Carbs: 19 g
Protein: 2 g
Sugar: 12 g

Both vitamins C and E are classified as antioxidants, and these two nutrients are available in abundance in bell peppers. In fact, a bell pepper has more vitamin C than an orange. This juice is a lovely vibrant color that might remind you of a sunrise, so all that vitamin C shouldn't be a surprise.

2 red bell peppers, cored and seeded
1 cup shredded and packed red cabbage
1 celery stalk with leaves
1 carrot
1 apple, cored

Feed the bell peppers through the juicer, followed by the cabbage and celery.

Feed the carrot and apple through the juicer.

Stir and pour the juice into 2 glasses. Drink immediately.

Serves 2

Spinach-Orange Juice

ANTI-CANCER ◆ DIGESTIVE HEALTH ◆ HEART HEALTH

Per Serving
Calories: 35
Fat: 0 g
Carbs: 10 g
Protein: 2 g
Sugar: 6 g

Spinach is one of the highest natural sources of the antioxidant lutein. It also contains high levels of beta-carotene and zeaxanthin. Some people avoid large quantities of spinach because it contains oxalic acid, which is thought to prevent the absorption of calcium and iron. Oxalic acid undergoes a change when cooked, which can create absorption issues, but raw spinach juice does not have this effect.

2 cups packed spinach
1 navel orange, peeled and sectioned
1 celery stalk with leaves
1 cucumber, halved lengthwise

Feed the spinach through the juicer, followed by the orange and celery.

Feed the cucumber through the juicer.

Stir and pour the juice into 2 glasses. Drink immediately.

Serves 2

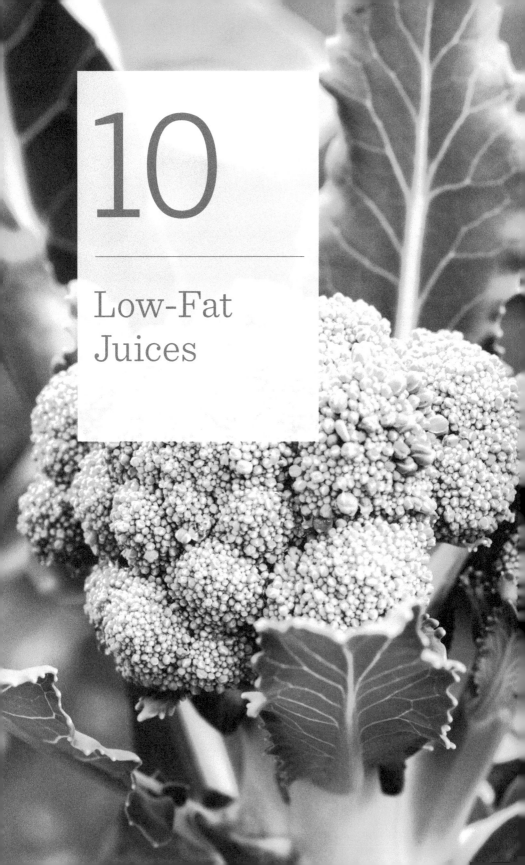

10

Low-Fat
Juices

RECIPES

Arugula-Celery Juice

ANTI-CANCER ◆ CLEANSE & DETOX ◆ HEART HEALTH

Per Serving
Calories: 24
Fat: 0 g
Carbs: 7 g
Protein: 1 g
Sugar: 5 g

Celery contains only 16 calories per cup, which makes it extremely valuable in creating low-calorie recipes like this one. Try using a Granny Smith apple to create a vibrant green juice; red apples will darken and dull the green from the arugula.

4 celery stalks with leaves
½ cup packed arugula
½ cucumber, halved lengthwise
½ apple, cored

Feed the celery through the juicer, followed by the arugula.

Feed the cucumber and apple through the juicer.

Stir and pour the juice into 2 glasses. Drink immediately.

Serves 2

Lovely Leafy Green Juice

ANTI-CANCER ◆ BONE & BLOOD HEALTH ◆ CLEANSE & DETOX

Per Serving
Calories: 60
Fat: 1 g
Carbs: 17 g
Protein: 3 g
Sugar: 9 g

Leafy greens of all varieties tend to be low in calories and high in nutrients. In this recipe you will find a combination of several leafy greens. This juice is a salad in a glass and just as flavorful.

2 romaine lettuce leaves
2 kale leaves
2 Swiss chard leaves
1 cup packed spinach
1 green-skinned pear, cored

Feed the lettuce, kale, and Swiss chard through the juicer.

Feed the spinach through the juicer, followed by the pear.

Stir and pour the juice into 2 glasses. Drink immediately.

Serves 2

Broccoli-Grapefruit Juice

ANTI-CANCER ◆ BONE & BLOOD HEALTH ◆ DIGESTIVE HEALTH

Per Serving
Calories: 162
Fat: 2 g
Carbs: 46 g
Protein: 14 g
Sugar: 21 g

Both broccoli and grapefruit are low-calorie ingredients that are high in nutrients. That means this recipe packs a double punch. This juice is tart with a hint of sweetness, depending on the flavor of your grapefruit.

1 pink grapefruit, peeled, sectioned, and seeded
1 head broccoli, chopped
1 celery stalk with leaves
1/2 lemon, peeled and seeded

Feed the grapefruit through the juicer, followed by the broccoli.

Feed the celery and lemon through the juicer.

Stir and pour the juice into a glass. Drink immediately.

Serves 1

Tangerine Green Juice

ANTI-CANCER ◆ BONE & BLOOD HEALTH ◆ HEART HEALTH

Per Serving
Calories: 42
Fat: 1 g
Carbs: 12 g
Protein: 4 g
Sugar: 4 g

Tangerines contain only 40 calories per fruit, whereas an orange can have 70 or more. Adding a tangerine to this green juice recipe gives it a hint of sweetness without greatly increasing the calorie count.

1 tangerine, peeled, seeded, and sectioned
1 celery stalk with leaves
2 cups fresh parsley
$\frac{1}{2}$ cup fresh cilantro
$\frac{1}{2}$ cup packed spinach

Feed the tangerine and celery through the juicer.

Feed the parsley, cilantro, and spinach through the juicer.

Stir and pour the juice into 2 glasses. Drink immediately.

Serves 2

Cranberry-Kale Juice

BRAIN HEALTH ◆ CLEANSE & DETOX ◆ HEART HEALTH

Per Serving
Calories: 40
Fat: 1 g
Carbs: 11 g
Protein: 3 g
Sugar: 2 g

Cranberries contain only 44 calories per cup and are naturally low in sugar. Combined with nutrient-rich kale, that makes this recipe a low-calorie wonder. You can use frozen cranberries in this juice if you thaw them completely first.

4 kale leaves
2 celery stalks with leaves
2 romaine lettuce leaves
1 cup cranberries
$^1/_2$ lemon, peeled and seeded

Feed the kale through the juicer, followed by the celery.

Feed the lettuce, cranberries, and lemon through the juicer.

Stir and pour the juice into 2 glasses. Drink immediately.

Serves 2

This juice has a very intense tart taste that will make your mouth water. The best way to juice cranberries is to pack your juicer chute with them rather than adding them in small amounts. If you want to cut the tartness a little, you can add a few fresh raspberries or strawberries to the mix.

Green Bell Pepper–Parsley Juice

ANTI-CANCER ◆ CLEANSE & DETOX ◆ HEART HEALTH

Per Serving
Calories: 35
Fat: 1 g
Carbs: 12 g
Protein: 2 g
Sugar: 5 g

Green bell peppers give this recipe a powerful nutrient profile, while fresh parsley lends a light, refreshing flavor. You can use either flat-leaf or curly leaf parsley for this recipe, depending on what you have in the fridge. Flat-leaf parsley has a more intense flavor, and both have the most flavor in the stems.

2 green bell peppers, cored and seeded
2 celery stalks with leaves
1 cucumber, halved lengthwise
1 cup fresh parsley
1 lemon, peeled, halved, and seeded

Feed the bell peppers through the juicer, followed by the celery and cucumber.

Feed the parsley through the juicer, followed by the lemon.

Stir and pour the juice into 2 glasses. Drink immediately.

Serves 2

Sweet Spinach-Basil Juice

ANTI-CANCER ◆ DIGESTIVE HEALTH ◆ HEART HEALTH

Per Serving
Calories: 32
Fat: 0 g
Carbs: 8 g
Protein: 1 g
Sugar: 7 g

Calorie for calorie, spinach has more nutrients than almost any other vegetable. Not only is it rich in nutrients, but it is a perfect low-calorie ingredient for juicing. It also creates a gorgeous deep-green juice that is a pleasure to drink.

2 cups packed spinach
1 cup packed fresh basil
1 apple, cored

Feed the spinach, basil, and apple through the juicer.

Stir and pour the juice into 2 glasses. Drink immediately.

Serves 2

Asparagus-Apple Juice

BONE & BLOOD HEALTH ◆ CLEANSE & DETOX ◆ HEART HEALTH

Per Serving
Calories: 47
Fat: 0 g
Carbs: 15 g
Protein: 2 g
Sugar: 9 g

Whether or not you are a fan of raw asparagus, you have to admit that it is a nutritional miracle. Incredibly high in folate, potassium, fiber, and vitamin K, it is surprisingly low in calories. Try to find stalks that are about the width of a pencil so they are tender without woody ends.

8 asparagus spears, trimmed
2 celery stalks with leaves
1 cup fresh cilantro
1 apple, cored
½ cucumber, halved lengthwise
½ lemon, peeled and seeded

Feed the asparagus through the juicer.

Feed the celery, cilantro, and apple through the juicer.

Feed the cucumber and lemon through the juicer.

Stir and pour the juice into 2 glasses. Drink immediately.

Serves 2

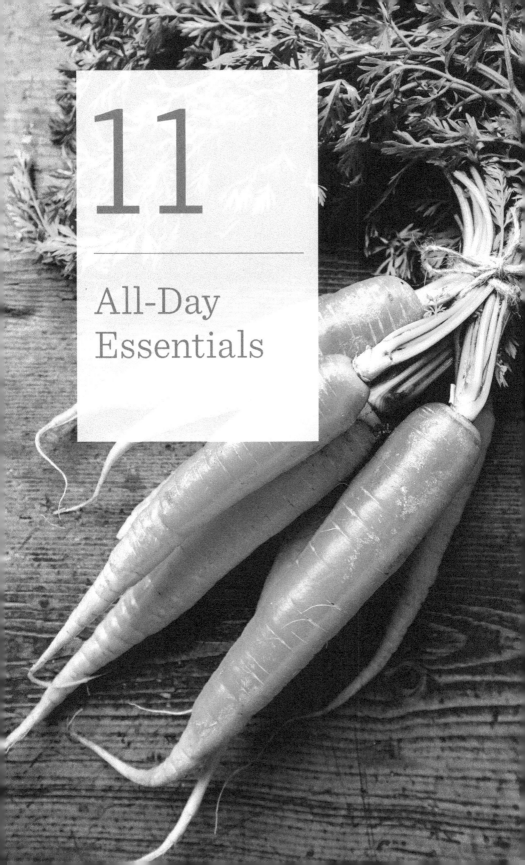

11

All-Day Essentials

RECIPES

Swiss Chard, Apple, and Fennel Swirl

ANTI-CANCER ◆ DIGESTIVE HEALTH ◆ HEART HEALTH

Per Serving
Calories: 99
Fat: 1 g
Carbs: 35 g
Protein: 5 g
Sugar: 7 g

Swiss chard has one of the broadest arrays of antioxidants of all vegetables. It also contains unique flavonoids called syringic acid that help regulate blood sugar. Fennel is loaded with vitamin C, and Golden Delicious apples are one of the most nutritious apple varieties.

2 cups packed Swiss chard (leaves and stems)
2 fennel bulbs
½ Golden Delicious apple, cored
½ teaspoon dried tarragon
½ teaspoon dried coriander

Feed the chard, fennel, and apple through the juicer.

Stir and pour the juice into a glass.

Stir in the tarragon and coriander. Drink immediately.

Serves 1

You can also use fresh herbs in this lovely juice for an even bolder taste. Simply add 1 teaspoon of chopped fresh tarragon and 1 teaspoon of chopped fresh cilantro with the Swiss chard. The best herbs for any healthful diet are ones you grow yourself, but organic products can also be a wonderful addition to your juices. Make sure you wash all herbs thoroughly because they grow close to the ground and can be contaminated with bacteria.

Herbed Turnip Greens and Tomato Splash

ANTI-CANCER ◆ CLEANSE & DETOX ◆ HEART HEALTH

Per Serving
Calories: 42
Fat: 1 g
Carbs: 13 g
Protein: 3 g
Sugar: 6 g

Turnip greens are loaded with calcium, folate, copper, manganese, and vitamins A, C, and K. They contain powerful antioxidants and anti-inflammatories and help lower LDL cholesterol. Turnip greens have a slightly bitter flavor, but when combined with tomatoes, celery, and oregano, they make for a flavorful juice.

2 cups packed turnip greens
2 tomatoes, quartered
2 celery stalks with leaves
1/2 teaspoon dried oregano

Feed the turnip greens, tomatoes, and celery through the juicer.

Stir and pour the juice into a glass.

Stir in the oregano. Drink immediately.

Serves 1

When purchasing tomatoes, look for the reddest ones, but watch for bruises and blemishes. The tomatoes should be soft, heavy, and yield to the touch. Smell is also an indicator of ripeness. Keep in mind that large tomatoes may be just as sweet and juicy as small ones. Store tomatoes at room temperature; refrigerating them will kill their flavor. If you have fresh oregano on hand, substitute dried oregano for 1 teaspoon of chopped fresh oregano.

Carrot, Lime, and Celery Cocktail

ANTI-CANCER ◆ DIGESTIVE HEALTH ◆ HEART HEALTH

Per Serving
Calories: 64
Fat: 3 g
Carbs: 10 g
Protein: 3 g
Sugar: 5 g

Flaxseed contains lignans, compounds that promote estrogen production. Research published in the British Journal of Nutrition *also suggests a link between lignans and lower body mass indexes (BMIs) in women. If you are taking a medication that slows blood clotting (anticoagulant or antiplatelet drugs), you should eliminate the flaxseed in this juice because it also slows blood clotting and can increase the chances of bruising and bleeding issues.*

¹⁄₄ **lime, peeled and seeded**
2 carrots
2 celery stalks with leaves
1 tablespoon ground flaxseed

Feed the lime, carrots, and celery through the juicer.

Stir and pour the juice into a glass.

Stir in the flaxseed. Drink immediately.

Serves 1

To prepare limes or any citrus fruit for juicing, cut a small sliver from the top and bottom to reveal the flesh. Sit one end on a flat surface and cut the exterior peel from top to bottom—just like peeling but with a knife.

Spinach, Cucumber, and Minty Beet Juice

ANTI-CANCER ◆ DIGESTIVE HEALTH ◆ HEART HEALTH

Per Serving
Calories: 83
Fat: 1 g
Carbs: 23 g
Protein: 5 g
Sugar: 11 g

Beets are a rich source of antioxidants and anti-inflammatories. They are also high in folate and contain manganese, copper, iron, magnesium, and phosphorus. The particular makeup of beet fiber makes it especially adept at fighting colon cancer and cardiovascular disease. As beets are very sweet, it takes only a small amount to add plenty of flavor.

$\frac{1}{2}$ beet with leaves (leaves optional)
2 cups packed spinach
1 tablespoon fresh mint leaves
2 cucumbers, halved lengthwise

Feed the beet through the juicer.

Turn off juicer and scoop 1 tablespoon of beet pulp from the pulp basket. Set aside.

Feed the spinach, mint leaves, and cucumbers through the juicer.

Add the reserved beet pulp to the juice.

Stir and pour the juice into a glass. Drink immediately.

Serves 1

Rutabaga, Peach, and Swiss Chard Sublime

ANTI-CANCER ❖ DIGESTIVE HEALTH ❖ HEART HEALTH

Per Serving
Calories: 118
Fat: 1 g
Carbs: 35 g
Protein: 5 g
Sugar: 21 g

Peaches have potassium and vitamins A and C, and according to the Journal of Medicinal Food, *they contain high amounts antioxidants known to fight cancer and help keep skin healthy. Peaches are a member of the rose family, which should be no surprise when you inhale its heady aroma. The sublime sweet taste of the peach is a perfect counterpart for the earthy flavor of the rutabaga.*

1 rutabaga, quartered and tops removed
1 peach, halved and pitted
1 cup packed Swiss chard (leaves and stems)
2 celery stalks with leaves

Feed the rutabaga and peach through the juicer, followed by the Swiss chard and celery.

Stir and pour the juice into a glass. Drink immediately.

Serves 1

Good peaches should be firm but yield to gentle pressure, and should not have any green on them. Avoid any bruised or overly soft peaches. The season for peaches varies depending on where they are grown, but they're usually best in August.

Zucchini, Arugula, and Radish Tonic

CLEANSE & DETOX ◆ DIGESTIVE HEALTH ◆ HEART HEALTH

Per Serving
Calories: 43
Fat: 1 g
Carbs: 10 g
Protein: 4 g
Sugar: 8 g

Zucchini is rich in vitamins B_6 and C and the mineral potassium. While arugula is used as a salad green, it actually belongs to the broccoli family and has many of the same vitamins, minerals, and cancer-fighting properties. Cilantro adds a pop of extra flavor to this juice.

2 zucchini, halved lengthwise
2 cups packed arugula
2 fresh parsley sprigs
2 fresh cilantro sprigs
2 radishes
1/4 teaspoon freshly ground black pepper

Feed the zucchini, arugula, parsley, cilantro, and radishes through the juicer.

Stir and pour the juice into a glass.

Stir in the pepper. Drink immediately.

Serves 1

Don't underestimate the power of a pinch or two of freshly ground black pepper. It is a great way to improve digestion. Pepper stimulates your taste buds to increase hydrochloric acid secretion, which helps your body digest proteins. For the best results, use whole peppercorn in a grinder.

Cinnamon and Sweet Potato Toddy

ANTI-CANCER ◆ DIGESTIVE HEALTH ◆ HEART HEALTH

Per Serving
Calories: 73
Fat: 0 g
Carbs: 20 g
Protein: 2 g
Sugar: 5 g

One cup of sweet potatoes provides fifteen times the vitamin A of a carrot. Sweet potatoes are also great sources for vitamins B6 and C, manganese, and copper. A spice that complements sweet potatoes, cinnamon may have antibacterial properties, according to a study in the Journal of Agricultural and Food Chemistry.

$^1\!/_2$ **sweet potato**
1 cup shredded and packed iceberg lettuce
1 teaspoon ground cinnamon

Feed the sweet potato and lettuce through the juicer.

Stir and pour the juice into a glass.

Stir in the cinnamon. Drink immediately.

Serves 1

Celery, Cantaloupe, and Cauliflower Blend

ANTI-CANCER ◆ DIGESTIVE HEALTH ◆ HEART HEALTH

Per Serving
Calories: 46
Fat: 0 g
Carbs: 12 g
Protein: 2 g
Sugar: 10 g

As a member of the cruciferous family, cauliflower is a powerhouse vegetable. High in vitamins C and K as well as folate, cauliflower is a well-known cancer fighter and friend of good cardiovascular health. Cantaloupe also abounds in vitamins A and C and adds a touch of sweetness to this detoxing juice.

¼ cantaloupe, peeled and seeded
1 cup cauliflower florets
2 fresh cilantro sprigs
2 celery stalks with leaves

Feed the cantaloupe and cauliflower through the juicer, followed by the cilantro and celery.

Stir and pour the juice into a glass. Drink immediately.

Serves 1

Cauliflower is a cruciferous vegetable, which means it is a wonderful tool for weight loss. It contains an array of nutrients that can support your goals by positively impacting the body. These vegetables stabilize blood sugar and hormones while boosting the metabolism, which is crucial for weight loss or maintenance.

Radishes, Corn, and Bell Pepper Blast

CLEANSE & DETOX ◆ DIGESTIVE HEALTH ◆ HEART HEALTH

Per Serving
Calories: 142
Fat: 2 g
Carbs: 36 g
Protein: 7 g
Sugar: 15 g

Radishes are high in vitamin C, and corn contains pantothenic acid, a B vitamin that excels at immune system support and converting food into energy for cells. Bell peppers are loaded with antioxidants, and even oregano is rich in phytonutrients and antibacterial agents.

2 radishes
1 cup fresh sweet corn
2 cucumbers, halved lengthwise
½ green bell pepper, cored and seeded
¼ teaspoon dried oregano

Feed the radishes, corn, cucumbers, and bell pepper through the juicer.

Stir and pour the juice into a glass.

Stir in the oregano. Drink immediately.

Serves 1

To cut kernels from the cob, first remove the husk and the silk. Hold the stem end of the shucked ear and rest the tip on the bottom of a large bowl. Using a paring knife, cut off the kernels and let them fall into the bowl. Be careful to cut just the kernels and not include any of the tough, inedible cob.

Pear, Purple Cabbage, and Tangerine Juice

ANTI-CANCER ◆ BONE & BLOOD HEALTH ◆ DIGESTIVE HEALTH

Per Serving
Calories: 77
Fat: 0 g
Carbs: 24 g
Protein: 2 g
Sugar: 16 g

Purple cabbage provides vitamins A and C and potassium as well as the rich color of this juice. If you are not a fan of the strong flavor of cabbage, you can lose the juice color and use milder Napa cabbage instead. Tangerine contributes additional vitamin C, and the pear melds all the flavors into a delicious, healthful blend.

½ pear, cored
1 cup shredded and packed purple cabbage
1 tangerine, peeled, seeded, and sectioned

Feed the pear, cabbage, and tangerine through the juicer.

Stir and pour the juice into a glass. Drink immediately.

Serves 1

Lemon, Swiss Chard, and Apple Swirl

BONE & BLOOD HEALTH ◆ DIGESTIVE HEALTH ◆ HEART HEALTH

Per Serving
Calories: 79
Fat: 1 g
Carbs: 23 g
Protein: 4 g
Sugar: 11 g

Despite their sweet taste, apples may actually help control blood sugar levels through their flavonoids. Gala is one of the most popular and mild-tasting varieties of apple. As an apple's fiber content is one of its best qualities, feel free to add some of the pulp back into the juice before drinking.

$\frac{1}{4}$ lemon, peeled and seeded
2 cups packed Swiss chard (leaves and stems)
2 cucumbers, halved lengthwise
$\frac{1}{4}$ Gala apple, cored

Feed the lemon and Swiss chard through the juicer, followed by the cucumbers and apple.

Stir and pour the juice into a glass. Drink immediately.

Serves 1

150

Spicy Radish and Carrot Punch

ANTI-CANCER ◆ CLEANSE & DETOX ◆ HEART HEALTH

Per Serving
Calories: 46
Fat: 1 g
Carbs: 15 g
Protein: 2 g
Sugar: 8 g

Except when consumed in large quantities, radishes are about as neutral in nutrients as a vegetable can be. But they do add a peppery kick to the fresh carrot, parsley, and celery flavors in this healthful drink. Try different types of radishes, including daikon, to get exactly the right taste for your palate.

2 radishes
2 carrots
2 fresh parsley sprigs
2 celery stalks with leaves

Feed the radishes and carrots through the juicer, followed by the parsley and celery.

Stir and pour the juice into a glass. Drink immediately.

Serves 1

Green Bell Pepper, Avocado, and Garlic Cocktail

ANTI-CANCER ◆ BONE & BLOOD HEALTH ◆ HEART HEALTH

Per Serving
Calories: 207
Fat: 21 g
Carbs: 17 g
Protein: 4 g
Sugar: 3 g

Avocados are rich in pantothenic acid (vitamin B$_5$), which is necessary for breaking down proteins, carbohydrates, and fats. Avocados also contain vitamin K, copper, and folate, and they help the body absorb carotenoids from other foods. Garlic adds selenium and a distinctive flavor, and a hot sauce like Tabasco adds some heat. The avocado and water is blended in a mixture to add some volume to the juice. Blending the avocado is recommended over mashing it with a fork so all lumps are eliminated and the texture is consistently smooth.

1 green bell pepper, cored and seeded
1 garlic clove
1 celery stalk with leaves
½ avocado, peeled and seeded
2 tablespoons spring water
Dash hot sauce

Feed the bell pepper, garlic, and celery through the juicer.

Stir and pour the juice into a glass.

Using a blender, combine the avocado and spring water.

Stir the avocado mixture and hot sauce into the juice. Drink immediately.

Serves 1

Peach, Rutabaga, and Ginger Swig

ANTI-CANCER ◆ DIGESTIVE HEALTH ◆ HEART HEALTH

Per Serving
Calories: 131
Fat: 1 g
Carbs: 39 g
Protein: 5 g
Sugar: 22 g

Ginger is known for its effectiveness in soothing digestive distress and nausea, but it also has antioxidant and anti-inflammatory properties. It adds a distinctive flavor to this unique combination of rutabaga and peach. Juice your ginger first so that the other ingredients push all the ginger through your juicer.

1 tablespoon peeled and sliced fresh ginger
1 peach, halved and pitted
2 cups shredded and packed romaine lettuce
1 rutabaga, quartered and tops removed

Feed the ginger and peach through the juicer, followed by the lettuce and rutabaga.

Stir and pour the juice into a glass. Drink immediately.

Serves 1

Rutabaga is a member of the cruciferous vegetable family, so it can help fight cancer. Since cancer-fighting properties are stronger in raw vegetables, juicing is the perfect way to enjoy them. This also means the health benefits of rutabagas are more effective when this vegetable is juiced in a masticating juicer that does not add any heat.

Zucchini, Spirulina, and Grape Booster

ANTI-CANCER ◆ BRAIN HEALTH ◆ HEART HEALTH

Per Serving
Calories: 138
Fat: 3 g
Carbs: 35 g
Protein: 14 g
Sugar: 11 g

Spirulina is a blue-green algae that contains many essential amino acids. Some people don't like spirulina's flavor, but combined with the tart grapes and fresh vegetables in this recipe, the flavor is quite subtle. Spirulina may be found in health food stores.

2 cups broccoli, stem included
2 zucchini, halved lengthwise
1 cup green grapes
2 celery stalks with leaves
1 tablespoon spirulina powder

Feed the broccoli, zucchini, grapes, and celery through the juicer.

Stir and pour the juice into a glass.

Stir in the spirulina powder. Drink immediately.

Serves 1

Apricot-Spinach Toddy

ANTI-CANCER ◆ CLEANSE & DETOX ◆ HEART HEALTH

Per Serving
Calories: 46
Fat: 1 g
Carbs: 13 g
Protein: 3 g
Sugar: 9 g

Apricots are high in beta-carotene, which helps protect against heart disease, and vitamin A for healthy vision. When you combine the rosy apricots with ginseng powder, you get a perfect mixture of tart and sweet. You should be able to find ginseng powder in most health stores.

3 apricots, halved and pitted
2 cups packed spinach
2 cups shredded and packed iceberg lettuce
½ teaspoon ginseng powder

Feed the apricots, spinach, and lettuce through the juicer.

Stir and pour the juice into a glass.

Stir in the ginseng powder. Drink immediately.

Serves 1

Bell Pepper and Purple Cabbage Splash

ANTI-CANCER ◆ DIGESTIVE HEALTH ◆ HEART HEALTH

Per Serving
Calories: 59
Fat: 1 g
Carbs: 18 g
Protein: 3 g
Sugar: 10 g

This juice combines the best of both the unripe (green) and ripe (red) versions of bell peppers. Bell peppers are high in folate and vitamins A, B6, and C, and they blend well with the mild cabbage and the fresh flavor of the celery. Make sure you always include the celery greens, because they contain five times more magnesium and calcium than the celery stalks.

1 green bell pepper, cored and seeded
1 red bell pepper, cored and seeded
2 cups shredded and packed purple cabbage
4 celery stalks with leaves

Feed the bell peppers, cabbage, and celery through the juicer.

Stir and pour the juice into a glass. Drink immediately.

Serves 1

Summer Squash and Arugula Punch

ANTI-CANCER ◆ BONE & BLOOD HEALTH ◆ BRAIN HEALTH

Per Serving
Calories: 41
Fat: 1 g
Carbs: 11 g
Protein: 4 g
Sugar: 7 g

Yellow summer squash is rich in vitamin C and excellent for juicing due to its mild flavor and high water content. Utilize young, fresh arugula leaves—they are milder—if you feel the combination of arugula and turmeric may prove too peppery. Make sure you stir the turmeric into this juice thoroughly, because it can float on top and create a film.

2 yellow summer squash
2 cups packed arugula
2 fresh parsley sprigs
2 celery stalks with leaves
½ teaspoon turmeric powder

Feed the squash, arugula, parsley, and celery through the juicer.

Stir and pour the juice into a glass.

Stir in the turmeric powder. Drink immediately.

Serves 1

Pineapple, Cauliflower, and Green Cabbage Blend

BONE & BLOOD HEALTH ◆ DIGESTIVE HEALTH ◆ HEART HEALTH

Per Serving
Calories: 102
Fat: 1 g
Carbs: 31 g
Protein: 6 g
Sugar: 18 g

Juicy, sweet pineapple dominates the flavor of this nutritious juice, which is why the other ingredients are all vegetables that are not sweet. The combination of greens, cauliflower, and pineapple load you up with vitamins A and C, B vitamins, copper, and manganese.

2 cups cauliflower florets
2 cups shredded and packed green cabbage
4 romaine lettuce leaves
1 cup diced pineapple

Feed the cauliflower and cabbage through the juicer, followed by the lettuce and pineapple.

Stir and pour the juice into a glass. Drink immediately.

Serves 1

Pineapple is a juicing ingredient that can cause some issues if you don't have the right juicer, because it is very fibrous. Centrifugal juicers can clog when you push pineapple through, so it is a good idea to push the pineapple through last. Make sure you remove the woody core before juicing this sweet fruit.

Plum Tomato, Greens, and Cayenne Blast

ANTI-CANCER ◇ CLEANSE & DETOX ◇ HEART HEALTH

Per Serving
Calories: 39
Fat: 1 g
Carbs: 11 g
Protein: 4 g
Sugar: 6 g

Tomatoes are rich in lycopene, a carotenoid that may lower your risk of stroke, according to researchers from Harvard Health Blog. *The Physicians Committee for Responsible Medicine also reported studies that have shown that lycopene may help prevent lung, stomach, and prostate cancer. With a variety of greens and herbs and a dash of cayenne, this juice bursts with flavor and health benefits.*

4 plum tomatoes or 8 cherry tomatoes
2 cups packed mustard greens
2 fresh parsley sprigs
2 fresh cilantro sprigs
2 celery stalks with leaves
½ teaspoon cayenne pepper

Feed the tomatoes, mustard greens, parsley, cilantro, and celery through the juicer.

Stir and pour the juice into a glass.

Stir in the cayenne pepper. Drink immediately.

Serves 1

Romaine and Zucchini Tonic

ANTI-CANCER ◆ CLEANSE & DETOX ◆ HEART HEALTH

Per Serving
Calories: 43
Fat: 1 g
Carbs: 11 g
Protein: 4 g
Sugar: 8 g

Romaine is high in nutrients and water content, and low in calories, making it an ideal juicing lettuce. Two cups of greens hold almost 300 percent of the recommended daily value of vitamin A, making it a powerful antioxidant. The dash of freshly ground black pepper provides a nice finish to this nutritious beverage.

2 cups shredded and packed romaine lettuce
2 zucchini, halved lengthwise
½ teaspoon freshly ground black pepper

Feed the romaine and zucchini through the juicer.

Stir and pour the juice into a glass.

Stir in the black pepper. Drink immediately.

Serves 1

This juice is for zucchini lovers because the taste of the romaine is lost in the stronger flavor of the summer squash. Zucchini is about 95 percent water, so it works very well in juicing recipes. You can try yellow zucchini as well in this recipe if you can't get green. Zucchini is a great tool to push the romaine leaves through the juicer, too.

Four Veggie and Blackberry Juice

ANTI-CANCER ◆ DIGESTIVE HEALTH ◆ HEART HEALTH

Per Serving
Calories: 74
Fat: 1 g
Carbs: 25 g
Protein: 4 g
Sugar: 13 g

This colorful drink is loaded with nutrition. The blackberries, carrots, and turnips are loaded with vitamins A, C, and K. They also provide plenty of B vitamins, magnesium, potassium, and manganese. This juice might have a strange dark color, but it is fresh tasting and sweet.

1 cup blackberries
2 carrots
1 turnip
1 cup shredded and packed romaine lettuce
2 celery stalks with leaves

Feed the blackberries, carrots, and turnip through the juicer.

Feed the lettuce and celery through the juicer.

Stir and pour the juice into a glass. Drink immediately.

Serves 1

Blackberries have the highest levels of antioxidants of any fruit. They are an aggregate fruit, which means they are part of a collection of smaller fruits called drupes. If blackberries aren't in season, substitute with blueberries, strawberries, cranberries, and/or raspberries.

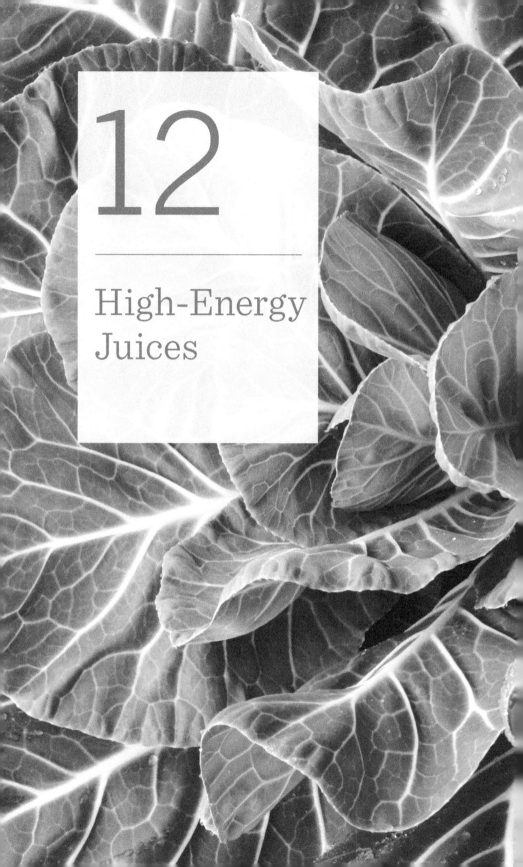

12

High-Energy Juices

RECIPES

Carrot, Apple, and Parsley Juice

ANTI-CANCER ◆ DIGESTIVE HEALTH ◆ HEART HEALTH

Per Serving
Calories: 115
Fat: 1 g
Carbs: 36 g
Protein: 3 g
Sugar: 22 g

Carrots are sometimes referred to as super roots because they contain so many nutrients. These vegetables help boost immune function and revitalize your body. You can juice them with the skin and greens still attached.

4 carrots
1 apple, cored
1 cup fresh parsley

Feed the carrots, apple, and parsley through the juicer.

Stir and pour the juice into a glass. Drink immediately.

Serves 1

Kale, Apple, and Broccoli Juice

ANTI-CANCER ◆ BONE & BLOOD HEALTH ◆ DIGESTIVE HEALTH

Per Serving
Calories: 131
Fat: 2 g
Carbs: 36 g
Protein: 8 g
Sugar: 17 g

Kale is not only a great source of natural energy, it is also loaded with antioxidant and anti-inflammatory benefits. You can use any variety of kale in this recipe, including green, red, purple, or curly. This is a good starter recipe for juices with kale, because you don't use too much and thus the flavor is milder.

2 kale leaves
2 broccoli stalks
1 apple, cored

Feed the kale, broccoli, and apple through the juicer.

Stir and pour the juice into a glass. Drink immediately.

Serves 1

Romaine, Carrot, and Lemon Juice

ANTI-CANCER ◆ CLEANSE & DETOX ◆ HEART HEALTH

Per Serving
Calories: 49
Fat: 1 g
Carbs: 16 g
Protein: 2 g
Sugar: 7 g

In addition to other essential nutrients, romaine lettuce contains about 136 micrograms of folate per serving. Folate helps regulate mood and also provides your body with a natural energy source.

3 carrots
3 fresh parsley sprigs
2 romaine lettuce leaves
$\frac{1}{2}$ lemon, peeled and seeded

Feed the carrots, parsley, lettuce, and lemon through the juicer.

Stir and pour the juice into a glass. Drink immediately.

Serves 1

The carrot in this juice provides the sweetness; try to find carrots less than six inches long, because they are sweeter than longer ones. Wash your carrots thoroughly and juice them without peeling them first, because many nutrients are found just under the skin. You don't want to peel away the health benefits.

166

Savvy Spinach-Lime Juice

ANTI-CANCER ◆ BRAIN HEALTH ◆ HEART HEALTH

Per Serving
Calories: 25
Fat: 0 g
Carbs: 10 g
Protein: 1 g
Sugar: 3 g

Spinach contains high levels of iron, which is a key element in energy production in the body. Enjoy this juice for a quick burst of energy. Spinach can be associated with allergies, though, so try not to exceed 16 ounces of spinach juice per day.

$\frac{1}{2}$ cup packed spinach
1 celery stalk with leaves
1 carrot
1 lime, peeled, halved, and seeded

Feed the spinach, celery, carrot, and lime through the juicer.

Stir and pour the juice into a glass. Drink immediately.

Serves 1

Celery can actually grow up to sixteen inches long, although you probably won't see that kind of height outside your own garden. Celery seems like a very humble vegetable, but its natural salty taste makes it a wonderful ingredient in juices. This natural sodium is safe for people who are salt sensitive, and it does not cause bloating, so it is appropriate for a weight-loss diet.

Celery-Cucumber Juice

BRAIN HEALTH ◆ DIGESTIVE HEALTH ◆ HEART HEALTH

Per Serving
Calories: 49
Fat: 1 g
Carbs: 13 g
Protein: 3 g
Sugar: 5 g

Both celery and cucumber are ideal for juicing because they each have such a high water content. They are also wonderful for slow-release energy, which stabilizes your blood sugar and appetite. Celery is also linked to lowering blood pressure.

1 (1-inch) piece fresh ginger, peeled
2 celery stalks with leaves
1 cucumber, halved lengthwise
1 handful fresh parsley

Feed the ginger and celery through the juicer, followed by the cucumber and parsley.

Stir and pour the juice into a glass. Drink immediately.

Serves 1

Wheatgrass-Celery Juice

ANTI-CANCER ◆ BONE & BLOOD HEALTH ◆ CLEANSE & DETOX

Per Serving
Calories: 65
Fat: 1 g
Carbs: 17 g
Protein: 13 g
Sugar: 9 g

Wheatgrass is a nutrient-rich grass that belongs to the wheat family. It contains a variety of vitamins and minerals that help raise energy levels and boost your immune system. You can also juice your wheatgrass separately in a wheatgrass juicer to avoid clogging your main juicer with fibrous plant material.

4 carrots
2 celery stalks with leaves
1 ounce fresh wheatgrass

Feed the carrots and celery through the juicer, followed by the wheatgrass.

Stir and pour the juice into a glass. Drink immediately.

Serves 1

Wheatgrass tastes like grass, which should not be a surprise. What might not be expected is the almost immediate reaction some people get when drinking this powerhouse ingredient. You can get nauseous and have diarrhea when not accustomed to wheatgrass, so start with small quantities until you are sure of the effect.

Lychee-Coconut Juice

ANTI-CANCER ◆ DIGESTIVE HEALTH ◆ HEART HEALTH

Per Serving
Calories: 80
Fat: 1 g
Carbs: 20 g
Protein: 2 g
Sugar: 13 g

Lychee is a juicy, nutritious white berry native to southern China. It contains a polyphenol called oligonol, which helps improve blood flow and reduce body weight. Make sure you do not skip the peeling step, because lychees have an inedible tough rind that will not juice.

20 lychees, peeled and seeded
1 cup sliced peaches
1 cup coconut water
Pinch ground cinnamon

In a blender, combine the lychees, peaches, and coconut water. Blend on high for 30 to 60 seconds, or until liquefied.

Strain the juice into 2 glasses and discard the solids.

Sprinkle the juice with ground cinnamon.
Drink immediately

Serves 2

This recipe is not actually a real juice when considering the definition being "from a juicer." However, you are discarding the solids, manually separating the pulp from juice, so this still qualifies as a juice drink. Make sure you use a medium-screen strainer, because peach juice is quite thick and will sometimes not go through a fine mesh.

Spinach-Almond Juice

BRAIN HEALTH ◆ DIGESTIVE HEALTH ◆ HEART DISEASE

Per Serving
Calories: 95
Fat: 6 g
Carbs: 11 g
Protein: 3 g
Sugar: 7 g

Almonds are an excellent source of protein and manganese, two nutrients that help keep energy flowing in your body. They also contain riboflavin, which helps support aerobic energy production. When not on a juice cleanse, you can use unsweetened almond milk instead of water in this recipe.

½ cup packed spinach
1 celery stalk with leaves
1 apple, cored
4 tablespoons raw almonds
Water to thin (optional)

Feed the spinach through the juicer, followed by the celery and apple.

In a blender, combine the juice and the almonds. Blend on high speed for 30 to 60 seconds, or until smooth.

Add water (if using) to thin the juice before serving.

Stir and pour the juice into 2 glasses. Drink immediately.

Serves 2

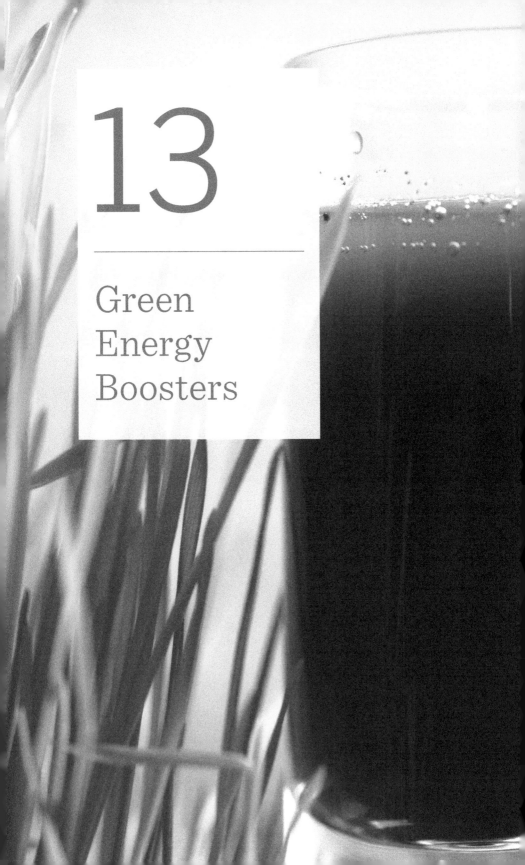

13

Green Energy Boosters

RECITES

Leafy Kale, Bok Choy, and Lime Tonic

ANTI-CANCER ◆ BONE & BLOOD HEALTH ◆ HEART HEALTH

Per Serving
Calories: 190
Fat: 3 g
Carbs: 41 g
Protein: 15 g
Sugar: 8 g

Baby bok choy provides plenty of vitamins A and C. Combined with the abundant vitamin K and minerals in the kale, this green juice is chock-full of nutrients. Bok choy has a very high water content, so it is an effective ingredient for juicing, especially when the other ingredients don't provide high juice yields.

1/4 lime, peeled and seeded
2 cups packed dinosaur kale (leaves and stems)
3 cups baby bok choy
2 cucumbers, halved lengthwise

Feed the lime and kale through the juicer, followed by the bok choy and cucumbers.

Stir and pour the juice into a glass. Drink immediately.

Serves 1

Wheatgrass, Peas, and Mint Cooler

BONE & BLOOD HEALTH ◆ BRAIN HEALTH ◆ CLEANSE & DETOX

Per Serving
Calories: 100
Fat: 1 g
Carbs: 19 g
Protein: 8 g
Sugar: 6 g

According to WebMD, wheatgrass contains the vitamins A, C, and E, minerals like iron and magnesium, and many of the amino acids needed for complete proteins. Wheatgrass juice is almost 50 percent protein, so it is often used in place of protein powder. You can find wheatgrass at natural food stores.

1 cup fresh wheatgrass greens or 1 tablespoon
  wheatgrass powder
½ cup spring water (if using fresh wheatgrass)
2 tablespoons fresh mint leaves
1 cup peas
1 celery stalk with leaves

If using fresh wheatgrass, crush it by hand with a mortar and pestle, then strain it into the spring water. Alternately, feed the wheatgrass through a wheatgrass juicer. Set aside.

Feed the mint, peas, and celery through the juicer.

Stir and pour the juice into a glass.

Stir in the wheatgrass juice (or powder, if using). Drink immediately.

Serves 1

Green Apple, Spinach, and Avocado Blend

ANTI-CANCER ◆ DIGESTIVE HEALTH ◆ HEART HEALTH

Per Serving
Calories: 157
Fat: 11 g
Carbs: 25 g
Protein: 3 g
Sugar: 14 g

Avocados have anti-inflammatories and antioxidants that promote cardiovascular health and relief from arthritic pain. Avocados cannot be juiced, so this drink will seem more like a smoothie than a juice. The spinach multiplies the green benefits of this drink, and the green apple adds a slightly tart bite.

1 Granny Smith apple, cored
2 cups packed baby spinach
¹⁄₂ avocado, peeled and pitted
¹⁄₂ cup spring water
Dash freshly ground black pepper

Feed the apple and spinach through the juicer.

Stir and pour the juice into a glass.

Using a blender, combine the avocado and spring water.

Stir the avocado mixture and black pepper into the juice. Drink immediately.

Serves 1

Radicchio, Celery, and Bell Pepper Punch

ANTI-CANCER ◆ BONE & BLOOD HEALTH ◆ CLEANSE & DETOX

Per Serving
Calories: 21
Fat: 0 g
Carbs: 6 g
Protein: 1 g
Sugar: 3 g

Radicchio, a purple and white Italian chicory, is loaded with vitamin K, which is essential for blood clotting. Cilantro is also incredibly rich in vitamin K, a serving containing about 250 percent of the daily recommended amount. Research from the Linus Pauling Institute at Oregon State University suggests that vitamin K intake can lower the risk of hip fractures among the elderly.

3/4 cup shredded and packed radicchio
4 celery stalks with leaves
2 fresh cilantro sprigs (optional)
1 green bell pepper, cored and seeded

Feed the radicchio and celery through the juicer, followed by the cilantro (if using) and bell pepper.

Stir and pour the juice into a glass. Drink immediately.

Serves 1

Green bell peppers are often overlooked next to their more flamboyant red, yellow, and orange counterparts. This is unfortunate because green bell peppers are a wonderful addition to juices. Make sure you purchase peppers with smooth, firm skins and that the peppers feel heavier than they look. This is a good indicator that they will yield a fair amount of juice.

Beet and Basil Cooler

BONE & BLOOD HEALTH ✦ CLEANSE & DETOX ✦ HEART HEALTH

Per Serving
Calories: 43
Fat: 1 g
Carbs: 13 g
Protein: 3 g
Sugar: 8 g

Basil is a rich source of vitamin K and contains enzymes that fight inflammation. The antioxidant properties of vitamin A and magnesium in basil are also good for heart health. The beet combines with the basil to make a colorful juice.

4 fresh parsley sprigs
½ beet
1 cup fresh basil
4 cups shredded and packed iceberg lettuce
Sparkling mineral water

Feed the parsley, beet, basil, and lettuce through the juicer.

Stir and pour the juice into a glass.

Top off the juice with the mineral water. Drink immediately.

Serves 1

Beet juice may be a great workout partner. A recent study at the University of Exeter's School of Sport and Health Sciences showed that drinking 2 cups of beet juice for six days increased physical performance. Researchers found the nitrates in beet juice helped people exercise up to 16 percent longer than usual. According to WebMD's director of nutrition, Kathleen M. Zelman, nitrates in beet juice help make exercise less tiring by reducing oxygen uptake.

Kohlrabi, Scallion, and Parsley Punch

ANTI-CANCER ◆ BONE & BLOOD HEALTH ◆ DIGESTIVE HEALTH

Per Serving
Calories: 60
Fat: 1 g
Carbs: 26 g
Protein: 7 g
Sugar: 11 g

The phytochemicals in kohlrabi have cancer-fighting benefits. Kohlrabi is a good source of vitamin C, containing more vitamin C than oranges. It also contains the minerals potassium, iron, copper, and phosphorus. Kohlrabi looks a bit like a turnip, but it is actually a cabbage.

2 light-green kohlrabi with leaves
2 scallions
4 fresh parsley sprigs
4 celery stalks with leaves

Feed the kohlrabi and scallions through the juicer, followed by the parsley and celery.

Stir and pour the juice into a glass. Drink immediately.

Serves 1

Scallions, also known as green onions or spring onions, are very high in vitamin K and high in vitamins A and B$_6$. They might seem like giant chives, but they are immature onions that do not develop into bulbs. You can juice both the white and green sections as long as you wash them very well.

Mustard Greens, Corn, and Celery Splash

CLEANSE & DETOX ◆ DIGESTIVE HEALTH ◆ HEART HEALTH

Per Serving
Calories: 300
Fat: 4 g
Carbs: 71 g
Protein: 20 g
Sugar: 26 g

Yellow corn has more carotenoids (a powerful antioxidant) than the white or blue varieties. Corn is high in protein and rich in vitamin B_6, magnesium, and iron. The green peas add manganese, copper, phosphorus, and vitamins B_1, C, and K.

2 cups packed mustard greens
2 cups fresh sweet corn
2 cups peas
1 celery stalk with leaves
Pinch salt

Feed the mustard greens and corn through the juicer.

Feed the peas and celery through the juicer

Stir and pour the juice into a glass.

Stir in the salt. Drink immediately.

Serves 1

Brussels Sprouts and Cayenne Cocktail

ANTI-CANCER ◆ CLEANSE & DETOX ◆ HEART HEALTH

Per Serving
Calories: 51
Fat: 1 g
Carbs: 15 g
Protein: 5 g
Sugar: 6 g

The glucosinolates and sulfur in Brussels sprouts support the body's natural detox systems and are believed to provide some cancer protection, according to The World's Healthiest Foods website. Brussels sprouts also have anti-inflammatory properties due to their omega-3 fatty acids. A bit of cayenne adds just a little heat to this juice.

2 cups Brussels sprouts
2 cups shredded and packed iceberg lettuce
4 celery stalks with leaves
Dash cayenne pepper

Feed the Brussels sprouts, lettuce, and celery through the juicer.

Stir and pour the juice into a glass.

Stir in the cayenne pepper. Drink immediately.

Serves 1

Cayenne pepper may spark your weight loss even more. Researchers at Purdue University have found that spicing your diet with cayenne pepper may decrease your appetite. You don't need much, either. Half a teaspoon in one daily meal may be enough to curtail cravings for unhealthful foods.

Collard Greens, Zucchini, and Beet Toddy

ANTI-CANCER ◆ BONE & BLOOD HEALTH ◆ HEART HEALTH

Per Serving
Calories: 66
Fat: 1 g
Carbs: 17 g
Protein: 5 g
Sugar: 11 g

As with other cruciferous vegetables, collard greens have strong cancer-fighting benefits. Few vegetables can compete with collards for vitamin K abundance. They also contain plenty of vitamins A and C, iron, and manganese, which are needed for bone and skin formation, protection from free radicals, and blood sugar stabilization.

1 cup packed collard greens
2 zucchini, halved lengthwise
½ beet
4 celery stalks with leaves

Feed the collard greens and zucchini through the juicer, followed by the beet and celery.

Stir and pour the juice into a glass. Drink immediately.

Serves 1

Parsley, Lime, and Radicchio Greenie

CLEANSE & DETOX • DIGESTIVE HEALTH • HEART HEALTH

Per Serving
Calories: 29
Fat: 0 g
Carbs: 8 g
Protein: 2 g
Sugar: 3 g

All too often parsley is added to plates as a garnish and discarded rather than eaten, but this powerful herb is a vitamin K star. It contains oils that impede tumor growth, folic acid needed for cell development and good cardiovascular health, and flavonoids that fight damaging oxidation. Chewing parsley is also a well-known breath freshener.

¼ lime, peeled and seeded
4 fresh parsley sprigs
3 cups shredded and packed radicchio
2 cups shredded and packed iceberg lettuce

Feed the lime and parsley through the juicer, followed by the radicchio and lettuce.

Stir and pour the juice into a glass. Drink immediately.

Serves 1

Radicchio is an often overlooked lettuce and is typically found only in vibrant red shreds in salad mixes. It has an interesting bitter taste and is a member of the chicory family. It is high in antioxidants, vitamin K, folic acid, iron, copper, and zinc.

Romaine, Kiwi, and Apple Cider Vinegar Blend

CLEANSE & DETOX • DIGESTIVE HEALTH • HEART HEALTH

Per Serving
Calories: 86
Fat: 1 g
Carbs: 25 g
Protein: 4 g
Sugar: 12 g

Apple cider vinegar can be used for everything from a hair conditioner and skin toner to a sunburn reliever and even a deodorant. It can also be used to ease indigestion, diarrhea, nasal congestion, and sore throats. Keep a bottle on hand for use during detoxification and cleansing diets.

2 cups shredded and packed romaine lettuce
1 kiwi, peeled and halved
2 cucumbers, halved lengthwise
1 tablespoon apple cider vinegar

Feed the romaine, kiwi, and cucumbers through the juicer.

Stir and pour the juice into a glass.

Stir in the vinegar. Drink immediately.

Serves 1

Mustard Greens and Wheatgrass Punch

ANTI-CANCER ◆ BONE & BLOOD HEALTH ◆ HEART HEALTH

Per Serving
Calories: 51
Fat: 0 g
Carbs: 9 g
Protein: 4 g
Sugar: 3 g

Like Brussels sprouts, mustard greens are rich in gluco-sinolates, which have cancer-fighting properties. They contain high levels of lutein, a component of vitamin A that is essential for healthful eyes and good vision. They have a lovely peppery taste, which can mask the rather strong taste of wheatgrass.

1 cup fresh wheatgrass greens or 1 tablespoon
   wheatgrass powder
½ cup spring water (if using fresh wheatgrass)
1 cup packed mustard greens
2 cups shredded and packed iceberg lettuce

If using fresh wheatgrass, crush it by hand with a mortar and pestle, then strain it into the spring water. Alternately, feed the wheatgrass through a wheatgrass juicer. Set aside.

Feed the mustard greens and lettuce through the juicer.

Stir and pour the juice into a glass.

Stir in the wheatgrass juice (or powder, if using). Drink immediately.

Serves 1

Green Protein Power Punch

BONE & BLOOD HEALTH ✦ DIGESTIVE HEALTH ✦ HEART HEALTH

Per Serving
Calories: 148
Fat: 2 g
Carbs: 19 g
Protein: 20 g
Sugar: 10 g

There are many types of protein powders on the market, but find one that is made from all vegetables, not dairy whey, for juice cleansing. Many protein powders are fortified with additional iron, vitamins, and minerals. Try several smaller containers of different brands, because there is a vast range of taste profiles among these products, and some can taste unpleasant if you are unfamiliar with protein powder.

2 cups shredded and packed iceberg lettuce
2 cucumbers, halved lengthwise
2 celery stalks with leaves
2 tablespoons vegetable protein powder

Feed the lettuce, cucumbers, and celery through the juicer.

Stir and pour the juice into a glass.

Stir in the protein powder. Drink immediately.

Serves 1

Arugula and Romaine Green Swirl

ANTI-CANCER ◆ BRAIN HEALTH ◆ DIGESTIVE HEALTH

Per Serving
Calories: 17
Fat: 1 g
Carbs: 5 g
Protein: 2 g
Sugar: 2 g

Lettuces make excellent bases for juices due to their high water content and mild flavors. Combining lettuces and celery provides a perfect beverage for taste-testing different spicy herbs and spices. Here, both ginseng and ginger are offered as options, but you may want to try experimenting with favorites of your own.

2 cups packed arugula
2 cups shredded and packed romaine lettuce
4 fresh parsley sprigs
4 celery stalks with leaves
1 tablespoon ginseng powder

Feed the arugula, romaine, parsley, and celery through the juicer.

Stir and pour the juice into a glass.

Stir in the ginseng powder. Drink immediately.

Serves 1

Pear, Parsley, and Celery Smash

BRAIN HEALTH ◆ CLEANSE & DETOX ◆ DIGESTIVE HEALTH

Per Serving
Calories: 41
Fat: 0 g
Carbs: 14 g
Protein: 1 g
Sugar: 9 g

The flavor of tarragon is similar to anise or licorice, so use only the coriander if that is not a flavor favorite. Tarragon has a long history as a medicinal herb used for toothaches, heart health, insomnia, and digestive problems. It is packed with nutrients, antioxidants, and minerals such as potassium.

$^1/_2$ **pear, cored**
4 fresh parsley sprigs
3 celery stalks with leaves
$^1/_4$ **teaspoon dried coriander**
$^1/_4$ **teaspoon dried tarragon**

Feed the pear, parsley, and celery through the juicer.

Stir and pour the juice into a glass.

Stir in the coriander and tarragon. Drink immediately.

Serves 1

Pears can actually be juiced whole, depending on the chute capacity or your juicer, even though their seeds contain cyanide. The amount of seeds found in a pear are only a tiny portion compared to the amount required to do harm. Since you are using only half your pear for this recipe, remember to brush the cut edge of the remaining half with a little lemon juice to prevent browning before you use it in your next juice.

Radicchio and Basil Green Juice

BONES & BLOOD HEALTH ◆ DIGESTIVE HEALTH ◆ HEART HEALTH

Per Serving
Calories: 98
Fat: 1 g
Carbs: 26 g
Protein: 6 g
Sugar: 11 g

Nearly all essential vitamins and minerals are found in basil, even if some are only in trace amounts. Vitamin K, which works with calcium, magnesium, and vitamin D to fortify bones, is the most plentiful. The best method for washing the grit from your basil is to submerge the leaves in a bowl of cold water and swirl them around. Then let the leaves float on the surface so the grit settles to the bottom of the bowl.

1 cup fresh basil
2 cups shredded and packed radicchio
4 fresh parsley sprigs
3 cucumbers, halved lengthwise

Feed the basil and radicchio through the juicer, followed by the parsley and cucumbers.

Stir and pour the juice into a glass. Drink immediately.

Serves 1

Fresh parsley should be kept in a plastic bag in the refrigerator. Sprinkling the parsley with some water or washing it without completely drying it before storing it will keep the parsley from wilting too fast. You can also place your parsley stems in a glass of water when storing it in the fridge, similar to arranging a bunch of flowers in a vase.

Radish and Arugula Refresher

ANTI-CANCER ◆ CLEANSE & DETOX ◆ DIGESTIVE HEALTH

Per Serving
Calories: 34
Fat: 1 g
Carbs: 9 g
Protein: 3 g
Sugar: 4 g

Slightly spicy, radishes may provide natural relief from sinus congestion during cold season. Radishes aid digestion, have detoxing properties, and possess the same cancer-fighting powers as broccoli and cabbage. Furthermore, their high water content makes them excellent juicing vegetables.

1 tablespoon peeled and sliced fresh ginger
4 radishes
4 cups packed arugula
2 cups shredded and packed iceberg lettuce

Feed the ginger and radishes through the juicer, followed by the arugula and lettuce.

Stir and pour the juice into a glass. Drink immediately.

Serves 1

Summer Squash and Kale Power Punch

ANTI-CANCER ◆ BONE & BLOOD HEALTH ◆ HEART HEALTH

Per Serving
Calories: 202
Fat: 4 g
Carbs: 32 g
Protein: 22 g
Sugar: 8 g

The skin and seeds of a summer squash are just as full of antioxidants as the flesh, and the whole squash makes for a mild-tasting, vitamin C–rich juice. Summer squash is also full of B vitamins, which are required to properly metabolize sugar. With the addition of protein powder and a radish, this drink is aptly named a power punch.

2 summer squash, halved lengthwise
2 cups packed dinosaur kale (leaves and stems)
4 celery stalks with leaves
1 radish
1 tablespoon vegetable protein powder

Feed the zucchini, kale, celery, and radish through the juicer.

Stir and pour the juice into a glass.

Stir in the protein powder. Drink immediately.

Serves 1

The radish in this juice can add quite a bit of heat, depending on how big it is and the type. Radishes contain a compound called isothiocyanate, which is also found in horseradish and wasabi. Taste your radishes before using them so you know exactly what you are adding to your juice. If you like heat, then toss in another radish for a truly fiery juice.

Cucumber, Spinach, and Tangerine Refresher

ANTI-CANCER ✦ CLEANSE & DETOX ✦ HEART HEALTH

Per Serving
Calories: 91
Fat: 1 g
Carbs: 25 g
Protein: 4 g
Sugar: 14 g

Cucumbers and spinach provide a fresh, springlike flavor to this juice. A tangerine adds to the already abundant vitamin C in this drink. Take the time to wash your spinach, because even prewashed products can have grit. The best way to juice baby spinach greens is to roll several leaves into a ball and push it through the juicer with bigger pieces of fruit or vegetable.

2 cucumbers, halved lengthwise
2 cups packed baby spinach
1 tangerine, peeled, seeded, and sectioned

Feed the cucumbers, spinach, and tangerine through the juicer.

Stir and pour the juice into a glass. Drink immediately.

Serves 1

Divine Green Juice

ANTI-CANCER ✦ DIGESTIVE HEALTH ✦ HEART HEALTH

Per Serving
Calories: 80
Fat: 1 g
Carbs: 22 g
Protein: 4 g
Sugar: 13 g

Quick and simple, yet full of fresh flavors, this recipe is nothing short of divine. There is enough kale in this recipe to reap health benefits but not enough to influence the taste very much. You can also substitute spinach for the kale—try about half a cup of packed leaves to make up the kale volume.

3 kale leaves
2 carrots
1 cucumber, halved lengthwise
1 green bell pepper, cored and seeded
1 cup fresh cilantro
1 apple, cored

Feed the kale and carrots through the juicer, followed by the cucumber and bell pepper.

Feed the cilantro and apple through the juicer.

Stir and pour the juice into 2 glasses. Drink immediately.

Serves 2

Swiss Chard–Spinach Juice

BRAIN HEALTH ◆ CLEANSE & DETOX ◆ HEART HEALTH

Per Serving
Calories: 12
Fat: 0 g
Carbs: 4 g
Protein: 1 g
Sugar: 2 g

Swiss chard is one of the greatest natural sources of vitamin K. One cup of Swiss chard contains more than 700 percent of your daily recommended value of vitamin K. This is a lovely green juice to enjoy at any time of the day.

2 celery stalks with leaves
1 carrot
2 cups packed Swiss chard (leaves and stems)
$\frac{1}{2}$ cup packed spinach

Feed the celery and carrot through the juicer, followed by the Swiss chard and spinach.

Stir and pour the juice into 2 glasses. Drink immediately.

Serves 2

Swiss chard has not had as much attention as its green counterparts, spinach and kale, but it is also packed with health-boosting nutrients. It is very high in vitamin K and an excellent source of vitamins A and C. Store the chard in the fridge in a sealed plastic bag without washing it first, because moisture will cause it to spoil faster.

Green Bean Sprouts Juice

BONE & BLOOD HEALTH ◆ DIGESTIVE HEALTH ◆ HEART HEALTH

Per Serving
Calories: 82
Fat: 1 g
Carbs: 24 g
Protein: 3 g
Sugar: 15 g

Bean sprouts are typically found in the organic section of the grocery store, sometimes with the prepared foods. Though you may not have noticed them in the past, after you try this recipe, you will be seeking them out. Make sure the bean sprouts are dry when you purchase them, because even a little moisture can make them slimy and inappropriate to juice.

2 cups bean sprouts
1 kale leaf
1 romaine lettuce leaf
1 cucumber, halved lengthwise
2 apples, cored
$\frac{1}{2}$ lemon, peeled and seeded

Pick through the bean sprouts, and discard any that are soft and brown.

Feed the bean sprouts through the juicer, followed by the kale and lettuce.

Feed the cucumber and apples through the juicer, followed by the lemon.

Stir and pour the juice into 2 glasses. Drink immediately.

Serves 2

Green Beet-Basil Juice

ANTI-CANCER ⬥ CLEANSE & DETOX ⬥ HEART HEALTH

Per Serving
Calories: 46
Fat: 0 g
Carbs: 15 g
Protein: 4 g
Sugar: 5 g

The combination of beet greens, basil, and fennel gives this recipe a unique flavor that you have to sip to believe. Beet greens are often difficult to find in the greens section, so save the ones that top your beets. Simply store them in a sealed plastic bag in your fridge.

2 cups chopped beet greens
2 cups fresh basil
1 beet, chopped
1 fennel bulb
½ cucumber, halved lengthwise

Feed the beet greens and basil through the juicer, followed by the beet, fennel, and cucumber.

Stir and pour the juice into 2 glasses. Drink immediately.

Serves 2

Dreamy Green Juice

ANTI-CANCER ◆ DIGESTIVE HEALTH ◆ HEART HEALTH

Per Serving
Calories: 138
Fat: 2 g
Carbs: 41 g
Protein: 7 g
Sugar: 21 g

This juice is so full of flavor and nutrients that you may find yourself dreaming about it. Broccoli can be juiced completely, from the stalk to the tightly packed florets. It does not produce a great yield, but the flavor is very intense.

1 head broccoli, chopped
2 romaine lettuce leaves
1 zucchini, halved lengthwise
2 pears, cored

Feed the broccoli and lettuce through the juicer, followed by the zucchini and pears.

Stir and pour the juice into 2 glasses. Drink immediately.

Serves 2

Broccoli is an excellent source of antioxidants as well as calcium and vitamins A, B6, C, E, and K. It is prized for its cancer-fighting properties, especially with respect to breast, cervical, lung, and colon cancer. Try to include this king of the cruciferous vegetables regularly in your diet.

Spicy Green Juice

BONE & BLOOD HEALTH ◆ CLEANSE & DETOX ◆ DIGESTIVE HEALTH

Per Serving
Calories: 20
Fat: 1 g
Carbs: 6 g
Protein: 2 g
Sugar: 2 g

When you think of juice, "spicy" probably isn't the first word that comes to mind. After trying this recipe, however, you will find yourself craving savory and spicy juices more often. They are a refreshing change from sweet blends.

2 Swiss chard leaves
4 cups shredded and packed romaine lettuce
1 celery stalk with leaves
1 jalapeño, seeded and halved
1 (1-inch) piece fresh ginger, peeled
1 garlic clove

Feed the Swiss chard and lettuce through the juicer, followed by the celery.

Feed the jalapeño and ginger through the juicer, followed by the garlic.

Stir and pour the juice into 2 glasses. Drink immediately.

Serves 2

Ginger, Celery, and Kale Juice

ANTI-CANCER ◆ BONE & BLOOD HEALTH ◆ DIGESTIVE HEALTH

Per Serving
Calories: 94
Fat: 1 g
Carbs: 26 g
Protein: 3 g
Sugar: 14 g

Loaded with vitamins and minerals, this recipe is just what you need to power up. If you don't like juices with a strong vegetable flavor, the apples in this recipe should sweeten it up for you. The ginger also cuts through the very green taste of kale.

1 (1-inch) piece fresh ginger, peeled
4 kale leaves
3 celery stalks with leaves
2 apples, cored
1 carrot

Feed the ginger and kale through the juicer, followed by the celery, apples, and carrot.

Stir and pour the juice into 2 glasses. Drink immediately.

Serves 2

Brilliant Brussels Sprouts Juice

ANTI-CANCER ◆ BONE & BLOOD HEALTH ◆ HEART HEALTH

Per Serving
Calories: 115
Fat: 1 g
Carbs: 34 g
Protein: 7 g
Sugar: 17 g

Don't hesitate to try this juice. Brussels sprouts add a unique flavor to this recipe that will surprise you. Many people don't like the taste of Brussels sprouts, but this is often due to overcooking this vegetable. Fresh Brussels sprouts juice might be a taste revelation.

10 Brussels sprouts
2 Swiss chard leaves
1 kale leaf
1 apple, cored

If the Brussels sprouts are still attached to a stalk, cut them off at the base of the bud.

Feed the Brussels sprouts through the juicer, followed by the Swiss chard and kale.

Feed the apple through the juicer.

Stir and pour the juice into a glass. Drink immediately.

Serves 1

Green Cucumber Lemonade

ANTI-CANCER ◆ CLEANSE & DETOX ◆ HEART HEALTH

Per Serving
Calories: 36
Fat: 1 g
Carbs: 11 g
Protein: 4 g
Sugar: 4 g

Leaving the peel on when juicing the lemon gives this recipe a distinctive flavor that is a good foil for the fresh greens. If you are leaving the peel on, purchase organic lemons to reduce your risk of pesticide exposure. This recipe is also lovely with limes.

2 kale leaves
2 romaine lettuce leaves
1 cucumber, halved lengthwise
8 asparagus spears, trimmed
1 lemon, halved and seeded

Feed the kale and lettuce through the juicer, followed by the cucumber and asparagus.

Feed the lemon through the juicer.

Stir and pour the juice into 2 glasses. Drink immediately.

Serves 2

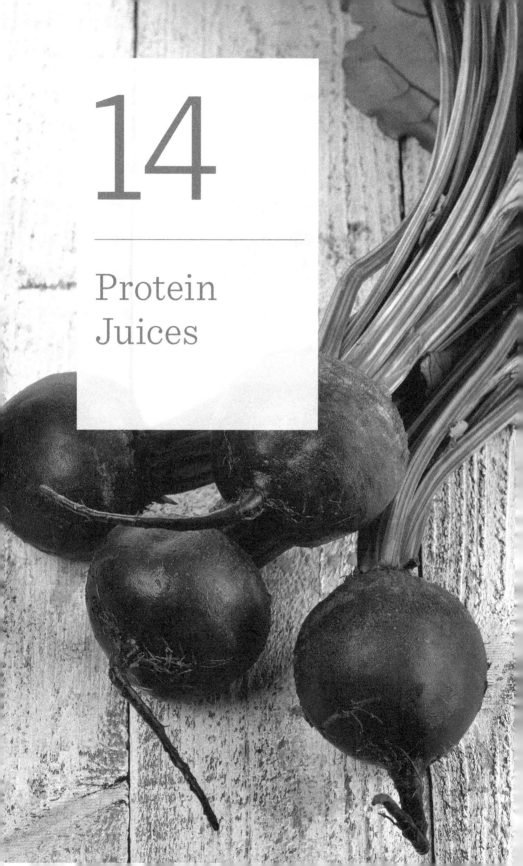

14

Protein
Juices

RECITES

Green Pea-Grape Juice

ANTI-CANCER ◆ DIGESTIVE HEALTH ◆ HEART HEALTH

Per Serving
Calories: 53
Fat: 1 g
Carbs: 16 g
Protein: 2 g
Sugar: 8 g

Green peas belong to the legume family and are an excellent source of vegetarian protein. One cup of peas contains almost 8 grams of protein, the same amount as a glass of milk. You can also use snow peas in this recipe.

1 cup seedless grapes
2 celery stalks with leaves
1 cup sugar snap peas
1 cup fresh cilantro
1 apple, cored

Feed the grapes and celery through the juicer, followed by the peas.

Feed the cilantro and apple through the juicer.

Stir and pour the juice into 2 glasses. Drink immediately.

Serves 2

Blueberry-Walnut Juice

ANTI-CANCER ◆ BRAIN HEALTH ◆ HEART HEALTH

Per Serving
Calories: 160
Fat: 10 g
Carbs: 20 g
Protein: 4 g
Sugar: 13 g

Raw nuts and seeds are rich in protein and heart-healthful fats. This recipe makes use of walnuts for a rich, nutty flavor. Try to find black walnuts, because they do not have the bitter taste associated with other types of walnuts.

½ cup packed spinach
1 cup blueberries
1 apple, cored
½ lemon, peeled and seeded
¼ cup raw walnuts

Feed the spinach through the juicer, followed by the blueberries.

Feed the apple through the juicer, followed by the lemon.

In a blender, combine the juice and walnuts. Blend on high speed for 30 to 60 seconds, or until smooth.

Pour the juice into 2 glasses. Drink immediately.

Serves 2

Sesame-Kale Juice

ANTI-CANCER ◆ BONE & BLOOD HEALTH ◆ HEART HEALTH

Per Serving
Calories: 150
Fat: 8 g
Carbs: 17 g
Protein: 5 g
Sugar: 7 g

Raw sesame seeds contain about 5 grams of protein per quarter cup. They are also a valuable source of mono-unsaturated fats. This recipe gives you an extra boost by adding a teaspoon of sesame oil to the finished juice.

6 kale leaves
2 celery stalks with leaves
1 romaine lettuce leaf
1 apple, cored
2 tablespoons raw sesame seeds
1 teaspoon sesame oil

Feed the kale, celery, lettuce, and apple through the juicer.

In a blender, combine the juice, sesame seeds, and sesame oil. Blend on high speed for 30 to 60 seconds, or until smooth.

Stir and pour the juice into 2 glasses. Drink immediately.

Serves 2

Broccoli-Carrot Juice

ANTI-CANCER ◆ BONE & BLOOD HEALTH ◆ DIGESTIVE HEALTH

Per Serving
Calories: 81
Fat: 1 g
Carbs: 25 g
Protein: 5 g
Sugar: 10 g

A single cup of broccoli contains about 8 grams of protein. That makes this recipe a wonderful protein boost after workouts or anytime. If you are using a centrifugal juicer, be aware that you will get very little juice out of your broccoli.

4 carrots
2 celery stalks with leaves
1 broccoli stalk

Feed the carrots, celery, and broccoli through the juicer.

Stir and pour the juice into a glass. Drink immediately.

Serves 1

Celery, Apple, and Hemp Juice

ANTI-CANCER ◆ BONE & BLOOD HEALTH ◆ DIGESTIVE HEALTH

Per Serving
Calories: 102
Fat: 3 g
Carbs: 21 g
Protein: 3 g
Sugar: 14 g

You may be familiar with hemp rope or even hemp clothing, but consuming hemp could be new to you. In this recipe you will see how hemp seeds can be a valuable addition to your diet. They can be found in the organic section of most major grocery stores.

4 celery stalks with leaves
2 apples, cored
2 romaine lettuce leaves
1 carrot
2 tablespoons ground hemp seed

Feed the celery through the juicer, followed by the apples.

Feed the lettuce and carrot through the juicer.

In a blender, combine the juice and the hemp seed. Blend on high speed for 30 to 60 seconds, or until smooth.

Stir and pour the juice into 2 glasses. Drink immediately.

Serves 2

Cucumber, Collard Greens, and Pistachio Juice

ANTI-CANCER ◆ BONE & BLOOD HEALTH ◆ HEART HEALTH

Per Serving
Calories: 146
Fat: 7 g
Carbs: 21 g
Protein: 3 g
Sugar: 11 g

While collard greens contain about 3 grams of protein per 100 grams, you get an extra boost of protein from the pistachios blended into this juice at the end. Try this juice as a pre- or post-workout boost.

4 collard greens leaves
2 carrots
1 cucumber, halved lengthwise
1 apple, cored
¼ cup shelled pistachios

Feed the collard greens and carrots through the juicer, followed by the cucumber and apple.

In a blender, combine the juice and the pistachios. Blend on high speed for 30 to 60 seconds, or until smooth.

Stir and pour the juice into 2 glasses. Drink immediately.

Serves 2

Bountiful Beet Juice

ANTI-CANCER ◆ CLEANSE & DETOX ◆ HEART HEALTH

Per Serving
Calories: 120
Fat: 1 g
Carbs: 37 g
Protein: 5 g
Sugar: 24 g

Beets are known for their nutritional value. What many people do not realize is that beet greens are just as healthful. One cup of beet greens contains 3 grams of protein. Try this recipe with golden beets as well for a sunshine-hued treat.

4 beets, peeled
2 cups chopped beet greens
1 apple, cored
½ cucumber, halved lengthwise
½ lemon, peeled and seeded

Feed the beets and greens through the juicer, followed by the apple and cucumber.

Feed the lemon through the juicer.

Stir and pour the juice into 2 glasses. Drink immediately.

Serves 2

Asparagus-Carrot Juice

ANTI-CANCER ◆ DIGESTIVE HEALTH ◆ HEART HEALTH

Per Serving
Calories: 114
Fat: 0 g
Carbs: 37 g
Protein: 3 g
Sugar: 22 g

Asparagus is not only rich in protein, it is also a good source of calcium, selenium, and vitamins A, C, and E. It has a strong taste that can be detected even when using only four spears. Try using an Asian pear in this recipe if you want your juice less sweet.

4 spears asparagus, trimmed
3 carrots
1 celery stalk with leaves
1 pear, cored

Feed the asparagus through the juicer.

Feed the carrots and celery through the juicer, followed by the pear.

Stir and pour the juice into a glass. Drink immediately.

Serves 1

When shopping for asparagus, get the greenest stalks possible, because the deeper the color, the more vitamin C the asparagus contains. Asparagus is a wonderful detoxifier and it can reduce water retention, which is great news when you are trying to lose weight.

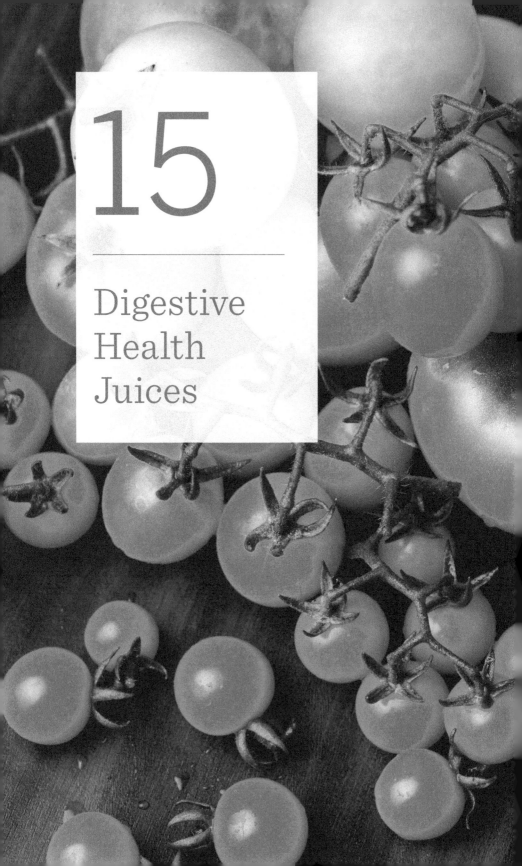

15

Digestive
Health
Juices

RECIPES

Zucchini-Cucumber Juice

CLEANSE & DETOX ◆ DIGESTIVE HEALTH ◆ HEART HEALTH

Per Serving
Calories: 151
Fat: 2 g
Carbs: 42 g
Protein: 7 g
Sugar: 22 g

Zucchini is not just a good ingredient for healthy digestion, it also helps lower cholesterol and stabilize blood sugar levels. With its high water content, zucchini acts as a mild diuretic to help detoxify the body. Try yellow or green zucchini in this recipe.

1 zucchini, halved lengthwise
½ cucumber, halved lengthwise
1 cup chopped kale
1 green-skinned pear, cored
½ lemon, peeled and seeded

Feed the zucchini through the juicer, followed by the cucumber.

Feed the kale, pear, and lemon through the juicer.

Stir and pour the juice into a glass. Drink immediately.

Serves 1

Lively Green Juice

BONE & BLOOD HEALTH ◆ BRAIN HEALTH ◆ DIGESTIVE HEALTH

Per Serving
Calories: 46
Fat: 1 g
Carbs: 10 g
Protein: 4 g
Sugar: 1 g

This combination of ingredients will wake up both you and your digestive system. Just to be sure, it has a bit of a kick from cayenne pepper. You can also add a piece of jalapeño pepper instead of cayenne pepper if you want a truly fiery juice.

1 (1-inch) piece fresh ginger, peeled
2 romaine lettuce leaves
2 kale leaves
½ cup fresh cilantro
½ cup fresh parsley
Pinch ground cayenne pepper

Feed the ginger, lettuce, and kale through the juicer, followed by the cilantro and parsley.

Stir and pour the juice into a glass.

Stir in the cayenne pepper. Drink immediately.

Serves 1

Artichoke, Celery, and Pear Juice

ANTI-CANCER ◆ CLEANSE & DETOX ◆ DIGESTIVE HEALTH

Per Serving
Calories: 113
Fat: 1 g
Carbs: 38 g
Protein: 5 g
Sugar: 18 g

Though artichokes may not look juicer-friendly, they actually juice quite well once you separate the leaves. This vegetable has been shown to improve digestion and to relieve irritable bowel syndrome. It can also prevent the buildup of toxins in the liver.

1 artichoke
2 celery stalks with leaves
1 plum tomato, halved
1 pear, cored

Cut off and discard the stem of the artichoke at the base of the bud. Remove and discard any tough or dry outer leaves.

Pull off the softer inner leaves of the artichoke and feed them through the juicer in small batches.

Chop the artichoke heart and feed it through the juicer.

Feed the celery, tomato, and pear through the juicer.

Stir and pour the juice into a glass. Drink immediately.

Serves 1

Raspberry-Flax Juice

CLEANSE & DETOX ✦ DIGESTIVE HEALTH ✦ HEART HEALTH

Per Serving
Calories: 81
Fat: 5 g
Carbs: 12 g
Protein: 5 g
Sugar: 3 g

High-fiber foods like raspberries and flaxseed help increase stool bulk, which aids in sweeping foods through the digestive tract more quickly. There usually is very little fiber in juices, so this juice has unique characteristics due to the flaxseed. A healthy digestive system is crucial when losing weight and keeping it off.

2 celery stalks with leaves
2 romaine lettuce leaves
1 cup raspberries
2 tablespoons ground flaxseed

Feed the celery, lettuce, and raspberries through the juicer.

In a blender, combine the juice and the flaxseed. Blend on high speed for 30 to 60 seconds, or until well combined.

Pour the juice into a glass. Drink immediately.

Serves 1

Papaya-Kale Juice

ANTI-CANCER ◆ DIGESTIVE HEALTH ◆ HEART HEALTH

Per Serving
Calories: 138
Fat: 1 g
Carbs: 39 g
Protein: 4 g
Sugar: 23 g

Papaya is a well-known digestive aid because it contains a natural enzyme that helps soothe the stomach and aid in the digestion of proteins. Papaya juices best when it is a bit under ripe. You can also use thawed frozen papaya if you can't find fresh.

½ cup chopped papaya, peeled
2 kale leaves
1 cup shredded and packed green cabbage
½ lemon, peeled and seeded

Feed the papaya through the juicer, followed by the kale, cabbage, and lemon.

Stir and pour the juice into a glass. Drink immediately.

Serves 1

Cucumber-Radish Juice

CLEANSE & DETOX ◆ DIGESTIVE HEALTH ◆ HEART HEALTH

Per Serving
Calories: 104
Fat: 1 g
Carbs: 33 g
Protein: 2 g
Sugar: 19 g

Foods that have a high water content are natural digestive aids because they help move foods through your digestive tract. Your body can't absorb fiber properly without water, which is another reason these foods are beneficial for digestive health.

3 radishes, greens included
1 cucumber, halved lengthwise
1 celery stalk with leaves
1 pear, cored

Feed the radishes and radish greens through the juicer, followed by the cucumber, celery, and pear.

Stir and pour the juice into a glass. Drink immediately.

Serves 1

Ginger-Beet Juice

ANTI-CANCER ◆ DIGESTIVE HEALTH ◆ HEART HEALTH

Per Serving
Calories: 80
Fat: 1 g
Carbs: 21 g
Protein: 3 g
Sugar: 12 g

Ginger not only helps relax the intestinal tract but it also helps reduce gas. In many cultures, ginger has been used as an herbal remedy to relieve nausea. A little goes a long way though, so don't use more than is specified in your recipes.

1 (1-inch) piece fresh ginger, peeled
3 kale leaves
1 beet, peeled and chopped
1 carrot
1 apple, cored

Feed the ginger, kale, and beet through the juicer, followed by the carrot and apple.

Stir and pour the juice into 2 glasses. Drink immediately.

Serves 2

Savory Tomato Juice

ANTI-CANCER ◆ BONE & BLOOD HEALTH ◆ DIGESTIVE HEALTH

Per Serving
Calories: 26
Fat: 0 g
Carbs: 8 g
Protein: 2 g
Sugar: 4 g

Tomatoes, due to their high water content, can aid digestion. But the real star of this recipe is cumin; it has been used medicinally to treat heartburn and as a digestive aid. It is also high in iron, which can boost your immune system and energy.

4 celery stalks with leaves
2 plum tomatoes, halved
1 red bell pepper, cored and seeded
1 cup fresh cilantro
1 lime, peeled, halved, and seeded
1 garlic clove
¼ teaspoon ground cumin

Feed the celery through the juicer, followed by the tomatoes, bell pepper, and cilantro.

Feed the lime halves and garlic through the juicer.

Stir the ground cumin into the juice.

Pour the juice into 2 glasses. Drink immediately.

Serves 2

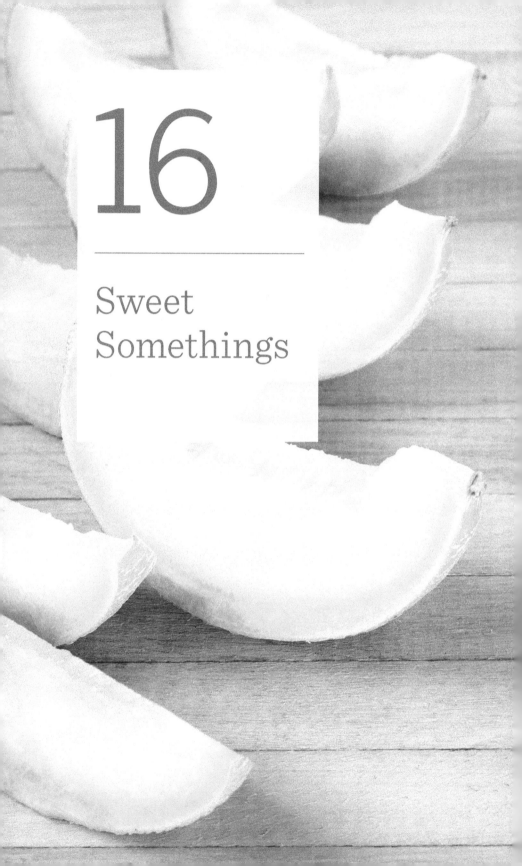

16

Sweet Somethings

RECIPES

Fig, Fennel, and Orange Cocktail

ANTI-CANCER ◆ DIGESTIVE HEALTH ◆ HEART HEALTH

Per Serving
Calories: 160
Fat: 1 g
Carbs: 53 g
Protein: 6 g
Sugar: 24 g

Sweet figs contain copper, magnesium, and potassium that may help control high blood pressure. If you have kidney or gallbladder issues, consult with your doctor before consuming too many figs. Figs are one of the most perishable fruits, so you will want to use them quickly after they ripen.

2 black mission or brown turkey figs, halved
2 fennel bulbs
1 navel orange, peeled and sectioned
2 celery stalks with leaves

Feed the figs and fennel bulbs through the juicer, followed by the orange and celery.

Stir and pour the juice into a glass. Drink immediately.

Serves 1

You might be wondering why you need to peel your navel orange in this recipe and all other citrus fruits you use in juicing recipes. The essential oils found in the peel add bitterness to the juice and can cause digestive issues. Lemon and lime peels can be left on if the fruit is organic and if you don't mind the extra-tart flavor.

Sweet Pear and Cauliflower Punch

ANTI-CANCER ◆ BONE & BLOOD HEALTH ◆ DIGESTIVE HEALTH

Per Serving
Calories: 117
Fat: 1 g
Carbs: 37 g
Protein: 5 g
Sugar: 21 g

Sweet pears are high in phytonutrients. According to a 2012 study published in the American Journal of Clinical Nutrition, *the skins and flesh of pears are especially high in the flavonoids anthocyanins, which are associated with a decreased risk of type 2 diabetes in women. Cauliflower delivers excellent amounts of vitamins C and K, and a study by the* Journal of Medicinal Chemistry *suggests the vegetable may help in cancer prevention.*

1 red-skinned pear, cored
1 head cauliflower with stalk, sectioned
2 cups shredded and packed iceberg lettuce

Feed the pear through the juicer. Turn off the juicer and scoop 1 tablespoon of pear pulp from the pulp basket. Set aside.

Feed the cauliflower and lettuce through the juicer.

Stir and pour the juice into a glass.

Stir in the reserved pear pulp. Drink immediately.

Serves 1

Apricot, Kale, and Honeydew Bubbly

BRAIN HEALTH ◆ DIGESTIVE HEALTH ◆ HEART HEALTH

Per Serving
Calories: 291
Fat: 2 g
Carbs: 76 g
Protein: 8 g
Sugar: 61 g

Apricots are a delicious source of vitamin A, which is essential to eye health and cell formation. Apricots are also a good source of vitamins C and E and potassium. Honeydew contributes a sweet flavor and potassium as well as vitamin B6, which helps protect against heart disease.

2 apricots, halved and pitted
1 cup packed dinosaur kale (leaves and stems)
1 cup honeydew melon, peeled, seeded, and diced
Sparkling mineral water

Feed the apricots, kale, and honeydew through the juicer.

Stir and pour the juice into a glass.

Top off the juice with the mineral water.
Drink immediately.

Serves 1

If you have trouble drinking enough plain water to stay well hydrated because it's so bland, switch to sparkling water. Not only do the bubbles jazz up the flavor, but sparkling water contains significant amounts of calcium. Some brands boast as much as 348 mg of calcium per liter, which is 44 percent of the recommended daily value for calcium.

Plum, Arugula, and Strawberry Juice

ANTI-CANCER ◆ BONE & BLOOD HEALTH ◆ DIGESTIVE HEALTH

Per Serving
Calories: 112
Fat: 1 g
Carbs: 32 g
Protein: 3 g
Sugar: 25 g

Despite their sweet taste, plums rate low on the glycemic index, which means they will have minimal impact on your blood sugar. Strawberries, which have been shown to help stabilize blood sugar, abound with vitamin C. Together, plums and strawberries make a sweet, nutritious treat.

4 red or purple plums, halved and pitted
1 cup sliced strawberries
2 cups packed arugula
2 celery stalks with leaves

Feed the plums and strawberries through the juicer, followed by the arugula and celery.

Stir and pour the juice into a glass. Drink immediately.

Serves 1

This juice will have a distinct strawberry taste despite the inclusion of several plums. Strawberries have a strong flavor, especially when ripe. They can be washed and popped into your juicer with the stems still attached.

Cantaloupe and Cranberry Swig

ANTI-CANCER ◆ DIGESTIVE HEALTH ◆ HEART HEALTH

Per Serving
Calories: 57
Fat: 1 g
Carbs: 17 g
Protein: 2 g
Sugar: 13 g

One cup of juicy, sweet cantaloupe has 98 percent of the recommended daily value of vitamin C. The unique antibacterial actions of proanthocyanidins found in cranberries give this fruit its power in fighting urinary tract infections. This is definitely not a sweet juice, because cranberries in their natural form are extremely tart and cantaloupe is not a very sweet melon. If you're not in the mood for a tart dessert, substitute blueberries for the cranberries.

1 cup cantaloupe, peeled, seeded, and cubed
$\frac{1}{2}$ cup cranberries
2 cups shredded and packed iceberg lettuce
2 celery stalks with leaves

Feed the cantaloupe and cranberries through the juicer, followed by the lettuce and celery.

Stir and pour the juice into a glass. Drink immediately.

Serves 1

Here's how to pick the best cantaloupe. First smell it: It should have a sweet, slightly musky scent. If it feels heavy for its size, the rind looks like raised netting, and the stem end gives slightly when pressed, you've found a good one.

Kiwi, Celery, and Banana Splash

BRAIN HEALTH ◆ DIGESTIVE HEALTH ◆ HEART HEALTH

Per Serving
Calories: 132
Fat: 1 g
Carbs: 38 g
Protein: 3 g
Sugar: 22 g

The combined sweetness of the banana and kiwis makes this juice taste like a dessert, but without added sugar and calories. These fruits also load you up on vitamins C and K as well as potassium and copper. Incorporating the banana provides some important fiber to lower LDL cholesterol and aid in digestion.

2 kiwis, peeled and halved
4 celery stalks with leaves
1 slightly under-ripe banana, peeled
½ cup unflavored coconut water

Feed the kiwis and celery through the juicer.

Stir and pour the juice into a glass.

Using a blender, combine the banana with the coconut water.

Stir the banana mixture into the juice.
Drink immediately.

Serves 1

When buying kiwis, look for firm ones. They'll ripen at room temperature in three to five days. Ripe kiwis have a pleasant, strawberry-like smell and are plump and slightly soft to the touch. Avoid ones with wrinkles, bruises, or soft spots.

Blueberry-Cucumber Punch

ANTI-CANCER ◆ BRAIN HEALTH ◆ DIGESTIVE HEALTH

Per Serving
Calories: 108
Fat: 1 g
Carbs: 31 g
Protein: 4 g
Sugar: 18 g

Blueberries rank among the highest of all antioxidant-rich foods. Not only are they sweet and delicious, studies have shown they help improve memory, steady blood sugar in people with type 2 diabetes, and are rich in manganese and vitamins C and K. To maximize their benefits, stick to organic, as nonorganic blueberries' nutrients are compromised.

1 cup blueberries
2 cucumbers, halved lengthwise
2 celery stalks with leaves

Feed the blueberries and cucumbers through the juicer, followed by the celery.

Stir and pour the juice into a glass. Drink immediately.

Serves 1

You will find cucumbers in many juicing recipes because they yield a high volume of juice and have a mild taste that combines well with a variety of ingredients. You do not have to peel them if they are English cucumbers. Plain field cucumbers often have wax on them, so you need to scrub them well or remove the peel. Cucumbers are also wonderful to use to push other produce through the juicer.

Bell Pepper, Carrot, and Tangerine Juice

ANTI-CANCER ◆ BONE & BLOOD HEALTH ◆ HEART HEALTH

Per Serving
Calories: 83
Fat: 1 g
Carbs: 23 g
Protein: 3 g
Sugar: 16 g

This is a truly lovely looking juice that bursts with color and a subtle orange fragrance. Red bell peppers are much higher in antioxidants than their unripened, green counterparts—and much sweeter. With the addition of carrot and tangerine, this satisfying juice is brimming with vitamins A and C.

2 red bell peppers, cored and seeded
1 carrot
1 tangerine, peeled, seeded, and sectioned
2 celery stalks with leaves

Feed the bell peppers and carrot through the juicer, followed by the tangerine and celery.

Stir and pour the juice into a glass. Drink immediately.

Serves 1

Remember to remove the stems from your red bell peppers because they should not be juiced. Red bell pepper is great for your skin and hair because it is high in vitamin E. It is also high in vitamin B_6, which helps promote a healthy nervous system.

Watermelon and Spinach Cooler

ANTI-CANCER ◆ DIGESTIVE HEALTH ◆ HEART HEALTH

Per Serving
Calories: 240
Fat: 2 g
Carbs: 63 g
Protein: 6 g
Sugar: 51 g

Although watermelon is higher in sugar than most fruits, the small amount in this juice is just enough to satisfy your sweet tooth without upsetting your blood sugar. Watermelon and spinach make this treat rich in vitamins A and C.

1 cup seedless watermelon cubes
2 cups packed spinach
4 celery stalks with leaves

Feed the watermelon, spinach, and celery through the juicer.

Stir and pour the juice into a glass. Drink immediately.

Serves 1

Put any cut-up watermelon in a bowl and refrigerate it; use it within two days. A piece of watermelon can be covered and refrigerated for three to four days. Watermelon can be juiced with the seeds, so simply cut off the rind and run it through your juicer.

The Dirty Dozen and Clean Fifteen

THE DIRTY DOZEN

The dirty dozen are fruits and vegetables the Environmental Working Group (EWG) has identified as being the most contaminated. When possible, choose organic when buying the produce on this list.

* Apples
* Bell peppers
* Celery
* Cherry tomatoes
* Cucumbers
* Grapes
* Hot peppers
* Nectarines (imported)
* Peaches
* Potatoes
* Spinach
* Strawberries

THE CLEAN FIFTEEN

The clean fifteen are nonorganic fruits and vegetables the EWG has identified as having the least amount of contamination. If you're watching your food budget, the clean fifteen are the best produce to buy nonorganic.

* Asparagus
* Avocados
* Cabbage
* Cantaloupe
* Eggplant
* Grapefruit
* Kiwis
* Mangoes
* Mushrooms
* Onions
* Papayas
* Peas (frozen)
* Pineapple
* Sweet corn
* Sweet potatoes

Appendix B Fruit and Vegetable Nutrition Charts

Fruits and vegetables are essential to effective weight loss. As previously established, the vitamins A and C found in produce are important for achieving and maintaining weight loss. Vitamin A helps strengthen your immune system and fight off possible infections while keeping your digestive system healthy and aiding in better nutrient absorption. Vitamin C helps you oxidize more fat during moderate exercise, and since exercising is a key component to any weight-loss plan, helping your body eliminate more fat while you work out is just plain smart.

Vegetables for Juicing

Percentages are based on the recommended daily values.

	Calories	Sugar	Vitamin A	Vitamin C
Arugula (1 cup)	4	0 g	5%	2%
Beets (1 cup)	58	9 g	1%	11%
Bell pepper (1 medium)	25	4 g	4%	190%
Bok choy (1 cup)	9	1 g	62%	52%
Broccoli (1 cup)	31	2 g	11%	135%
Brussels sprouts (1 cup)	38	2 g	13%	125%
Cabbage (1 cup)	16	0 g	1%	30%
Carrots (1 medium)	30	5 g	110%	10%
Cauliflower (1 cup)	28	2 g	0%	92%

Vegetables for Juicing *continued*

	Calories	Sugar	Vitamin A	Vitamin C
Celery (2 medium stalks)	15	2 g	10%	15%
Collard greens (1 cup)	11	0 g	48%	21%
Corn, sweet (1 cup)	132	5 g	0%	17%
Cucumber (1 medium)	30	3 g	12%	30%
Kale (1 cup)	33	0 g	206%	134%
Kohlrabi (1 cup)	36	4 g	1%	140%
Lettuce, iceberg (1 cup)	10	1 g	7%	3%
Lettuce, romaine (1½ cups)	15	1 g	130%	6%
Mustard greens (1 cup)	15	1 g	118%	65%
Parsley (1 cup)	22	1 g	101%	133%
Parsnips (1 cup)	100	6 g	0%	38%
Radicchio (1 cup)	9	0 g	0%	5%
Radish (1 cup)	18	2 g	0%	28%
Rutabaga (1 cup)	50	8 g	0%	58%
Scallions (1 cup)	32	2 g	20%	31%
Spinach (1 cup)	7	0 g	56%	14%
Sugar snap peas (¾ cup)	20	2 g	4%	10%
Summer squash (½ medium)	20	2 g	6%	30%
Sweet potato (1 medium)	100	7 g	120%	30%
Swiss chard (1 cup)	7	0 g	44%	18%
Tomatoes (1 medium)	25	3 g	20%	40%
Turnip Greens (1 cup)	25	1 g	140%	30%
Turnips (1 cup)	36	5 g	0%	46%
Zucchini (1 large)	3	0 g	2%	9%

Fruits for Juicing

Percentages are based on the recommended daily values.

	Calories	Sugar	Vitamin A	Vitamin C
Apple (1 large)	130	25 g	2%	8%
Apricot (1 cup)	74	14 g	60%	26%
Avocado (1 cup)	240	1 g	4%	25%
Banana (1 medium)	110	19 g	2%	8%
Blackberries (1 cup)	62	7 g	6%	50%
Blueberries (1 cup)	84	15 g	2%	24%
Cantaloupe (1 cup)	60	14 g	120%	108%
Cranberries (1 cup)	50	4 g	1%	24%
Figs (1 large)	47	10 g	2%	2%
Grapefruit (½ medium)	60	11 g	35%	100%
Grapes (¾ cup)	90	20 g	0%	2%
Guava (1 cup)	112	15 g	21%	628%
Honeydew (1 cup)	64	14 g	2%	53%
Kiwis (2 medium)	90	13 g	2%	240%
Lemon (1 medium)	15	2 g	0%	35%
Lime (1 medium)	20	0 g	0%	35%
Nectarine (1 medium)	60	11 g	8%	15%
Orange (1 medium)	80	14 g	2%	130%
Papaya (1 cup)	55	8 g	31%	144%
Peach (1 medium)	60	13 g	6%	15%
Pear (1 medium)	100	16 g	0%	10%
Pineapple (1 cup)	82	16 g	2%	131%
Plums (2 medium)	70	16 g	8%	160%

Fruits for Juicing *continued*

	Calories	Sugar	Vitamin A	Vitamin C
Raspberries (1 cup)	64	5 g	1%	54%
Strawberries (1 cup)	49	7 g	0%	149%
Tangerine (1 medium)	50	9 g	6%	45%
Watermelon (2 cups)	80	1 g	30%	25%

Appendix C Measurement Conversions

Oven Temperatures

Celsius (C)	Fahrenheit (F)
120	250
150	300
180	355
200	400
220	450

Volume Equivalents

Metric	Imperial (approximate)
20 ml	½ fl oz
60 ml	2 fl oz
80 ml	3 fl oz
125 ml	4½ fl oz
160 ml	5½ fl oz
180 ml	6 fl oz
250 ml	9 fl oz
375 ml	13 fl oz
500 ml	18 fl oz
750 ml	1½ pints
1 liter	1¾ pints

Weight Equivalents

Metric	Imperial (approximate)
10 g	⅓ oz
50 g	2 oz
80 g	3 oz
100 g	3½ oz
150 g	5 oz
175 g	6 oz
250 g	9 oz
375 g	13 oz
500 g	1 lb
750 g	1⅔ lb
1 kg	2 lb

Cup and Spoon Conversions

Metric	Imperial (approximate)
5 ml	1 teaspoon
20 ml	1 tablespoon
60 ml	¼ cup
80 ml	⅓ cup
125 ml	½ cup
160 ml	⅔ cup
180 ml	¾ cup
250 ml	1 cup

Resources

HEALTHFUL FOOD DOCUMENTARIES

A juice cleanse can leave you feeling cleaner, more energized, and motivated to change your eating habits. For further inspiration and education on what to eat, what to avoid, and how your food choices impact your long-term health, watch any or all of these acclaimed documentaries. The more you know about food and how it gets to your plate, the more likely you are to make the right dietary choices.

Fat, Sick & Nearly Dead

Australian Joe Cross takes a sixty-day journey across the United States while following a fruit and vegetable juice fast, with Joel Fuhrman, Nutrition Research Foundation's director of research, serving as his health advisor. By the end, Cross loses about 100 pounds on his all-juice diet and is healthy enough to stop taking all his medications.

Food, Inc.

Do you really know where your food comes from? And better still, why does it matter? This film focuses on corporate farming in the United States and takes the stance that the country's agribusiness produces food that is mostly unhealthful, environmentally harmful, and abusive of both animals and employees. There is a particular focus on the harmful and dangerous industrial production of chicken, beef, and pork as well as grains and vegetables like corn and soybeans. There is also an emphasis on common and questionable business practices, such as food-labeling regulations, the dependency on contaminated food because of its low cost, and the heavy use of pesticides and fertilizers.

Food Matters

Can food heal? This documentary, directed by James Colquhoun and Carlo Ledesma, tries to answer that question by focusing on how a selective diet can treat a range of health conditions—diabetes, cancer, heart disease, and depression—and how it may even trump traditional medicine.

Forks Over Knives

Similar to *Food Matters,* this documentary investigates how a healthful, low-fat, plant-based diet can combat a variety of diseases. The film is based on the research of physician Caldwell Esselstyn and professor of nutritional biochemistry T. Colin Campbell and their work on the China-Cornell-Oxford Project. Their findings conclude that the typical Western diet of processed, animal-based and dairy foods is actually the cause of coronary disease, diabetes, obesity, and cancer, and that eating healthfully can save your life.

Vegucated

Vegan diets can be hard to follow, and this film highlights the ongoing challenges and obstacles of people who opt to eat an animal-free diet. The stars are three ordinary meat-eating New Yorkers who try to follow a vegan diet for six weeks.

References

Academy of Nutrition and Dietetics. "Do You Have Tips for Buying Fresh Fruits and Veggies?" Accessed February 16, 2014. http://www.eatright.org/Public/content. aspx?id=6442451954.

Adkins, Clarissa. "Can Cinnamon Help You Lose Weight?" LiveStrong.com. Last modified August 16, 2013. http://www. livestrong.com/article/199161-can-cinnamon-help-you-lose-weight/.

Ballentine, Rudolph. *Diet and Nutrition: A Holistic Approach.* Honesdale, PA: Himalayan Institute Press, 2007.

Bechtel, Jonathan. "The Beginner's Guide to Juice Fasting." *Living Green Magazine.* May 21, 2012. http://livinggreenmag. com/2012/05/21/food-health/the-beginners-guide-to-juice-fasting/.

Bella NutriPro. "Top 10 Reasons to Juice." Accessed December 2, 2013. http://www.nutriprojuicer.com/articles/top-10-reasons-to-juice.

Boston University Medical Center. "Diet High in Vegetables and Fruit Associated with Less Weight Gain in African-American Women." ScienceDaily. May 20, 2011. www.sciencedaily.com/releases/2011/05/110520104834.htm.

Braverman, Eric R. *Younger (Thinner) You Diet: How Understanding Your Brain Chemistry Can Help You Lose Weight, Reverse Aging, and Fight Disease.* New York: Rodale, 2009.

CBS News. "Vitamin E May Help Treat Liver Disease." CBSNews.com. April 29, 2010. http://www.cbsnews.com/news/vitamin-e-may-help-treat-liver-disease/.

Diets.MD. "Can Diet Shakes and Meal Replacement Really Help You Lose Weight?" Accessed February 16, 2014. http://www.diets.md/reviews.php?title=can-diet-shakes-and-meal-replacements-really-help-you-lose-weight.

Ding, Sara. "What to Expect When You Juice Fast?" Juicing-for-Health.com with Sara Ding. Accessed February 16, 2014. http://juicing-for-health.com/joy-of-juicing/juice-fasting/what-to-expect-when-juice-fast.html.

Elsevier Health Sciences. "Is Long-Term Weight Loss Possible after Menopause?" ScienceDaily. August 28, 2012. www.sciencedaily.com/releases/2012/08/120828093238.htm.

Everyday Juicer. "Step 6: Spice It Up." Accessed February 16, 2014. http://www.everydayjuicer.com/step-6-spice-it-up/.

EWG (Environmental Working Group). "EWG's 2013 Shopper's Guide to Pesticides in Produce." Accessed April 2, 2014. http://www.ewg.org/foodnews/summary.php.

Examiner.com. "Drink a Salad: A Quick Guide to Juice Cleansing." June 23, 2011. http://www.examiner.com/article/drink-a-salad-a-quick-guide-to-juice-cleansing.

FDA (US Food and Drug Administration). "Raw Produce: Selecting and Serving It Safely." Food Facts. Last modified August 12, 2013. http://www.fda.gov/Food/ResourcesForYou/Consumers/ucm114299.

Food for Life Cancer Project. "How Lycopene Helps Protect against Cancer." Physicians Committee for Responsible Medicine. Accessed March 14. 2014. http://pcrm.org/health/cancer-resources/diet-cancer/nutrition/how-lycopene-helps-protect-against-cancer.

Fred Hutchinson Cancer Research Center. "Mid-morning Snacking May Sabotage Weight-Loss Efforts." ScienceDaily. November 28, 2011. www.sciencedaily.com/releases/2011/11/111128132716.htm.

Gamonski, William. "Cauliflower the Head of the Cruciferous Vegetable Family." *Life Extension Magazine*. January 2013. https://www.lef.org/magazine/mag2013/jan2013_Cauliflower-the-Head-of-the-Cruciferous-Vegetable-Family_01.htm.

Gerbstadt, Christine. *Doctor's Detox Diet: The Ultimate Weight Loss Solution*. Sarasota, FL: Nutronics Health Publishing, 2012.

Gittleman, Ann Louise. *The Fast Track Detox Diet: Boost Metabolism, Get Rid of Fattening Toxins, Jump-Start Weight Loss, and Keep the Pounds Off for Good*. New York: Morgan Road Books, 2006.

Glynn, Mark. "Healthy Eating Tips: How Cumin Can Aid in Weight Loss." Oswego Patch. August 7, 2012. http://oswego.patch.com/groups/dr-mark-glynns-blog/p/bp--healthy-eating-tips-how-cumin-can-aid-in-weight-loss.

Godman, Heidi. "Lycopene-Rich Tomatoes Linked to Lower Stroke Risk." *Harvard Health Blog*. October 10, 2012. http://www.health.harvard.edu/blog/lycopene-rich-tomatoes-linked-to-lower-stroke-risk-201210105400.

Guzman, Anne. "Can Beet Juice Instantly Improve Your Endurance?" Accessed March 6, 2014. http://www.active.com/cycling/articles/can-beet-juice-instantly-improve-your-endurance.

Haas, Elson M. "Nutrition Program for Fasting." Healthy.net. Accessed April 2, 2014. http://www.healthy.net/Health/Article/Nutritional_Program_for_Fasting/1996.

Haas, Elson M., with Buck Levin. *Staying Healthy with Nutrition: The Complete Guide to Diet and Nutritional Medicine.* rev. ed. Berkeley, CA: Celestial Arts, 2006.

Hackett, Jolinda. "Easy Homemade Vegetable Soup." About.com. Accessed February 16, 2014. http://vegetarian.about.com/od/soupsstewsandchili/r/Easy-Homemade-Vegetable-Soup.htm.

Higdon, Jane and Victoria J. Drake. "Vitamin K." Linus Pauling Institute. Last modified December 19, 2011. http://lpi.oregonstate.edu/infocenter/vitamins/vitaminK/.

Hofmekler, Ori. "Cruciferous Indoles for a Healthy Estrogen Metabolism." Mahler's Aggressive Strength. Accessed February 16, 2014. http://www.mikemahler.com/online-library/articles/nutrition-programs/cruciferous-indoles-for-healthy-estrogen-metabolism.html.

Institute of Food Technologists. "Spicing Up Food Can Make Up for Missing Fat." ScienceDaily. July 15, 2013. www.sciencedaily.com/releases/2013/07/130715134640.htm.

Johnston, C. S. "Strategies for Healthy Weight Loss: From Vitamin C to the Glycemic Response." *Journal of the American College of Nutrition* 24, no. 3 (June 2005): 158–65. http://www.ncbi.nlm.nih.gov/pubmed/15930480.

Lifespan. "Study Shows Keys to Successful Long-Term Weight Loss Maintenance." ScienceDaily. January 6, 2014. www.sciencedaily.com/releases/2014/01/140106115351.htm.

Lipman, Frank. "What Do You Mean by Detox?" Care2. September 19, 2010. http://www.care2.com/greenliving/what-do-you-mean-by-detox.html.

Lissandrello, Maria. "Healing Foods: Papaya." *Vegetarian Times.* Accessed March 14, 2014. http://www.vegetariantimes.com/article/healing-foods-papaya/.

Living Greens. "Benefits." Accessed December 3, 2013. http://www.livinggreensjuice.com/benefits-of-juicing-s/1824.htm.

Mattes, Richard. "Soup and Satiety." *Physiology and Behavior* 83 (2005): 739–47. http://www.indiana.edu/~abcwest/pmwiki/CAFE/Soup%20and%20satiety.pdf.

Mayo Clinic Staff. "Water: How Much Should You Drink Every Day." Mayo Clinic. October 12, 2011. http://www.mayoclinic.org/water/ART-20044256.

MedlinePlus. "Diet—Chronic Kidney Disease." National Institutes of Health. Last modified September 21, 2011. http://www.nlm.nih.gov/medlineplus/ency/article/002442.htm.

Melancon, Merritt. "UGA Study: Produce Sometimes Better Frozen than Fresh." *Online Athens: Athens Banner-Herald*. December 7, 2013. http://onlineathens.com/health/2013-12-07/uga-study-produce-sometimes-better-frozen-fresh.

Morisset, Anne-Sophie, Simone Lemieux, Alain Veilleux, Jean Bergeron, S. John Weisnagel, and André Tchernof. "Impact of a Lignan-Rich Diet on Adiposity and Insulin Sensitivity in Post-Menopausal Women." *British Journal of Nutrition* 102. no. 2 (July 2009): 195–200. doi:10.1017/S0007114508162092.

Moss, Michael. "Are Nuts a Weight-Loss Aid?" *New York Times*. December 17, 2013. http://www.nytimes.com/2013/12/18/dining/are-nuts-a-weight-loss-aid.html?_r=0.

National Institutes of Health. "Vitamin D." US Department of Health and Human Services. Accessed March 16, 2014. http://ods.od.nih.gov/factsheets/VitaminD-HealthProfessional/.

National Kidney Foundation. "Low Vitamin D Levels Linked to Early Signs of Kidney Disease." Accessed March 16, 2014. http://www.kidney.org/news/newsroom/nr/Low-Vitamin-D-Levels-Linked-to-Early-Signs-of-KD.cfm.

Nutrition Source. "Vegetables and Fruits: Get Plenty Every Day." Harvard School of Public Health. Accessed February 16, 2014. http://www.hsph.harvard.edu/nutritionsource/vegetables-full-story/.

Preventive Medicine Center. "Why Unprocessed Grains?" Accessed February 16, 2014. http://www.thepmc.org/2009/12/why-unprocessed-grains/.

Purdue University. "Reasonable Quantities of Red Pepper May Help Curb Appetite, Study Suggests." ScienceDaily. April 26, 2011. www.sciencedaily.com/releases/2011/04/110425173902.htm.

Renal Business Today. "Low Vitamin D Levels Linked to Early Signs of Kidney Disease." June 27, 2013. http://www.renalbusiness.com/news/2013/06/low-vitamin-d-levels-linked-to-early-signs-of-kidney-disease.aspx.

Rossato, S. B., C. Haas, M. C. do Raseira, J. C. Moreira, and J. A. Zuanazzi. "Antioxidant Potential of Peels and Fleshes of Peaches from Different Cultivars." *Journal of Medicinal Food* 12, no. 5 (October 2009): 1119–26. http://www.ncbi.nlm.nih.gov/pubmed/19857078.

Sass, Cynthia. "Planning a Detox or Juice Cleanse? 5 Dos and Don'ts." Health.com. July 18, 2013. http://news.health.com/2013/07/18/planning-a-detox-or-juice-cleanse-5-dos-and-donts/.

Shan, Bin, Yi-Zhong Cai, John D. Brooks, and Harold Corke. "Antibacterial Properties and Major Components of Cinnamon Stick (*Cinnamomum burmannii*): Activity against Foodborne Pathogenic Bacteria." *Journal of Agricultural and Food Chemistry* 55, no. 14 (2007): 5484–90. http://pubs.acs.org/doi/abs/10.1021/jf070424d.

Temasek Polytechnic. "Benefits of Low Glycemic Index Foods." Glycemic Index Research Unit. Accessed February 16, 2014. http://www-as.tp.edu.sg/asc_home/asc_aboutus/ asc_aboutus_ce/asc_aboutus_ce_giru/asc_microsite_ benefits_of_low_glycemix_index_foods.htm.

University of Granada. "Melatonin Might Help Control Weight Gain and Prevent Heart Disease Associated with Obesity." ScienceDaily. April 28, 2011. www.sciencedaily.com/ releases/2011/04/110428092501.htm.

Valliant, Melissa. "Do Juice Cleanses Work? 10 Truths about the Fad." *Huffington Post*. Last modified November 11, 2013. http://www.huffingtonpost.ca/2012/03/22/do-juice-cleanses-work_n_1372305.html.

WebMD. "Grapefruit Juice: Is It Affecting Your Medicine?" Hypertension/High Blood Pressure Center. Last modified October 30, 2013. http://www.webmd.com/hypertension-high-blood-pressure/guide/grapefruit-juice-and-medication.

WebMD. "Wheatgrass." Accessed March 14, 2014. http://www. webmd.com/vitamins-supplements/ingredientmono-1073-wheatgrassaspx?activeIngredientId=1073&activeIngredient Name=wheatgrass.

Wedick, Nicole M., An Pan, Aedín Cassidy, Eric B. Rimm, Laura Sampson, Bernard Rosner, Walter Willett, Frank B. Hu, Qi Sun, and Robert M. van Dam. "Dietary Flavonoid Intake and Risk of Type 2 Diabetes in US Men and Women." *American Journal of Clinical Nutrition* (April 2012). Published electronically February 22, 2012. doi:10.3945/ ajcn.111.028894.

Worldometers. "Overweight People in the World—Definition, Sources, and Methods." Accessed December 3, 2013. http:// www.worldometers.info/weight-loss/.

World's Healthiest Foods. "What's New and Beneficial about Brussels Sprouts." Accessed March 14, 2014. http://www.whfoods.com/genpage.php?tname=foodspice&dbid=10.

Zelman, Kathleen M. "The Truth about Beetroot Juice." WebMD. Accessed March 6, 2014. http://www.webmd.com/food-recipes/features/truth-about-beetroot-juice.

Zelman, Kathleen M. "The Truth about Kale." WebMD. Accessed March 6, 2014. http://www.webmd.com/food-recipes/features/the-truth-about-kale.

Zeratsky, Katherine. "I Like to Drink Grapefruit Juice but Hear That It Can Interfere with Some Prescription Medications. Is That True?" Mayo Clinic Expert Answers. http://www.mayoclinic.org/food-and-nutrition/expert-answers/faq-20057918.

Ingredient Index

Index

Ingram Content Group UK Ltd.
Milton Keynes UK
UKHW050238210323
418837UK00008B/68